Acrobats of the Gods

Marie-Louise von Franz, Honorary Patron

**Studies in Jungian Psychology
by Jungian Analysts**

Daryl Sharp, General Editor

Acrobats
of the Gods

Dance and Transformation

JOAN DEXTER BLACKMER

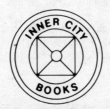

To my mother, Jeannette Pruyn Reed, who danced me into life, and to family and friends, students and teachers with whom I have danced over the years.

Canadian Cataloguing in Publication Data

Blackmer, Joan Dexter, 1931-
    Acrobats of the gods: dance and transformation

(Studies in Jungian psychology by Jungian analysts; 39)

Bibliography: p.
Includes index.

ISBN 0-919123-38-4

1. Dancing—Psychological aspects.   2. Mind and body.
3. Dance therapy.   4. Jung, C.G. (Carl Gustav), 1875-1961.
I. Title.   II. Series.

RC489.D3B53 1989   616.89'1655   C89-094359-1

INNER CITY BOOKS
Box 1271, Station Q, Toronto, Canada M4T 2P4
Telephone (416) 927-0355

Honorary Patron: Marie-Louise von Franz.
Publisher and General Editor: Daryl Sharp.
Senior Editor: Victoria Cowan.

INNER CITY BOOKS was founded in 1980 to promote the
understanding and practical application of the work of C.G. Jung.

Front Cover: Dancing Shiva (12th cent. bronze, South India).

Back Cover: Sara Yarborough in Alvin Ailey's "The Lark Ascending."
    (Photo by Kenn Duncan, in Olga Maynard, *Judith Jamison:
    Aspects of a Dancer,* Doubleday, 1982.)

Index by Daryl Sharp

Printed and bound in Canada by Webcom Limited

Contents

See final pages for descriptions of other Inner City Books

Illustration Credits

Page 8 from Reynold Higgins, *Minoan and Mycenaean Art,* New York, Praeger, 1967.

Pages 12, 59, 63, 77, from C.G. Jung, *Psychology and Alchemy,* CW 12.

Pages 17, 21, from John Martin, *John Martin's Book of the Dance,* New York, Tudor Publishing Co., 1963.

Pages 22, 73, from Erich Neumann, *The Great Mother* (Bollingen Series XLVII), Princeton, Princeton University Press, 1963.

Page 25 from Ben Martin, *Marcel Marceau: Maitre Mime,* Montreal, Editions Optimum, 1978.

Pages 27, 49, from Suzanne Gordon, *Off Balance: The Real World of Ballet,* New York, Pantheon, 1983.

Page 30 from Margaret Hebblethwaite, *Motherhood and God,* London, Geoffrey Chapman, 1984.

Page 33 from Barbara Morgan, *Martha Graham: Sixteen Dances in Photographs,* Dobbs Ferry, NY, Morgan and Morgan, 1980.

Page 36 (top) from Curt Sachs, *World History of the Dance,* New York, W.W. Norton, 1937.

Pages 36 (bottom), 108, author's collection.

Page 38 from Houser, *Dionysos and His Circle,* Fogg Art Museum, Harvard University, 1979.

Pages 39, 87, 98, 101, 104, from LeRoy Leatherman, *Martha Graham: Portrait of the Lady as an Artist,* New York, Alfred A. Knopf, 1966.

Pages 40, 55, from Leonardo da Vinci, *Drawings,* New York, Dover, 1980.

Page 43 from *Stones, Bones and Skin: Ritual and Shamanic Art,* Toronto, The Society for Art Publications, 1977.

Pages 45, 64, 71, from James Klosty, *Merce Cunningham,* New York, Dutton, 1975.

Pages 57, 83 (right), from Fritz Kahn, *The Human Body,* New York, Random House, 1965.

Page 67 from Joseph H. Mazo, *Prime Movers: The Makers of Modern Dance in America,* New York, Wm. Morrow, 1977.

Page 75 from Olga Maynard, *Judith Jamison: Aspects of a Dancer,* New York, Doubleday and Co., 1982.

Pages 80, 92, from John Percival, *Modern Ballet,* New York, Harmony Books, 1980.

Page 83 (left) from Brendon Lehane, *The Power of Plants,* New York, McGraw-Hill, 1977.

Page 94 from Martha Graham and Dance Co., 1949 program.

Page 107 courtesy Museum of Fine Arts, Boston; purchased by contribution.

Page 113 from Anatole Chujoy and P.W. Manchester, *The Dance Encyclopedia,* New York, Simon and Schuster, 1967.

There is a vitality, a life-force, an energy, a quickening that is translated through you into action and because there is only one of you in all of time, this expression is unique. And if you block it, it will never exist . . . . The world will not have it.
—Martha Graham.

Sport puts an exceptional valuation on the body, and this tendency is emphasized still further in modern dancing. . . . The fascination of the psyche brings about a new self-appraisal, a reassessment of our fundamental human nature. We can hardly be surprised if this leads to a rediscovery of the body after its long subjugation to the spirit—we are even tempted to speak of the body's revenge upon the spirit.
—C.G. Jung, *Modern Man in Search of a Soul.*

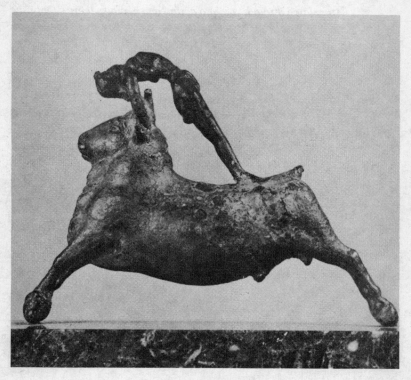

Bull and acrobat.
(Bronze, Crete, 16th cent.; British Museum, London)

1
Introduction

In recent years there has been an enormous upsurge of interest and participation in physical activity. Physical culture in one form or another is pursued with an almost compulsive intensity—the collective seems to be gripped by a passion to sculpt and strengthen the body. Jogging, aerobics, tennis, skiing and swimming are all the rage; so, too, are "magic" diets and fitness programs. Foods, vitamins, herbs and exercises seem to be a new pharmacopoeia, potentially curing everything from cancer and heart disease to the common cold.

The psychological tree now sprouts physical branches: bio-energetics, sensory awareness, primal scream, bio-feedback, *t'ai chi,* yoga, massage of both gentle and violent sorts—these are but a few of the many "new discoveries." Flesh seems to be seeking a more conscious place in human life. After two thousand years of repression, physicality is straining at its chains.

Indeed, the energy of the body and the instincts embedded therein must be enormous, else the Christian era would not have had to spend such a vast amount of effort to contain it. "Asceticism," notes Jung, "occurs whenever the animal instincts are so strong that they need to be violently exterminated."[1]

Yet we cannot simply shake our fists at Christianity's suppression of animal instincts, for this very suppression has been responsible for the development of rational consciousness—the hallmark of Western culture. Jung speaks to this:

> The Christian idea of sacrifice is symbolized by the death of the human being and demands a surrender of the whole man—not merely a taming of his instincts, but a total renunciation of them and a disciplining of his specifically human, spiritual functions for the sake of

---

[1] *Symbols of Transformation,* CW 5, par. 119n. (CW refers throughout to *The Collected Works of C.G. Jung)*

9

a spiritual goal beyond this world. This ideal is a hard schooling which cannot help alienating man from his own nature and, to a large degree, from nature in general. The attempt, as history has shown, was entirely possible and led in the course of a few centuries to a development of consciousness which would have been quite out of the question but for this training.[2]

The time seems ripe, now that we have worked so hard to develop our mental capacities, to differentiate and train the flesh, to tame it rather than renounce it. Then its energy and instinctive wisdom, which in repression have not been absent but simply autonomous and often angry, can be joined to consciousness.

We may now be ready to use the tools of reason and consciousness, fashioned by the act of Christian renunciation, to explore the matter from which we spring; not by examining a deadened body, inanimate subject of the dissection table, but with feeling and caring, even with admiration and affection, allowing it to breathe, permitting life to flow through it consciously.

With our heads reconnected to our bodies (and thus to our hearts), we can strive not for perfection of the spirit but rather, with Eros, for greater awareness of the continuity and wholeness of the body-spirit spectrum.

It seems to me that all this interest in matter, in *physis,* is part and parcel of a new activation of an evolving feminine archetype, one whose roots lie in matter but whose branches reach to a feminine variety of spirit. Here I am concerned with the roots.

Indeed, it seems that the branches have been split from the roots of the feminine tree. In "Answer to Job," Jung describes how the incarnation of Christ was "queered" by Yahweh's careful exclusion of human flesh from his plans. Mary was immaculate, untainted by original sin. The dominant masculine ideal of perfection kept her pure:

> Her freedom from original sin sets Mary apart from mankind in general, whose common characteristic is original sin and therefore the

---

2 Ibid., par. 674.

need of redemption. . . . By having these special measures applied to her, Mary is elevated to the status of a goddess and consequently loses something of her humanity: she will not conceive her child in sin, like all other mothers, and therefore he also will never be a human being, but a god. . . . To my knowledge at least, no one has ever perceived that this queers the pitch for a genuine Incarnation of God, or rather, that the Incarnation was only partially consummated. Both mother and son are not real human beings at all, but gods.[3]

In 1950 Pope Pius XII proclaimed as dogma that the much-loved but still immaculate Mary had been taken up into heaven, *in her body,* to be the bride of her son. This was the culmination of a centuries-old "deep longing in the masses for an intercessor and mediatrix who would at last take her place alongside the Holy Trinity and be received as 'Queen of Heaven and Bride at the heavenly court.' "[4] The divinity of the feminine principle, and matter itself, was recognized.

The concomitant material reverberations of this, its roots on earth and in the human psyche, have released energies which cause celibate priests to marry and beget fleshly children, nuns to leave the convent, women to seek liberation and all of us increasingly to be concerned with the conservation and preservation of Mother Nature's resources.

The consequences within the feminine psyche are illustrated by the following dream. The dreamer was a woman of forty-five, much concerned with the changes which seemed to be taking place within herself and within the feminine archetype.

I am in an enclosed medieval city square. In the center is a small park with green grass. While in one of the ground-floor shops that surround the square, I hear a person pacing the floor above me.

I am told that a woman named Mary has been kept a prisoner by her father in the room above for many years, perhaps all of her life, but now she is going to be allowed to descend and walk around the square.

---

3 *Psychology and Religion,* CW 11, par. 626.
4 Ibid., par. 748.

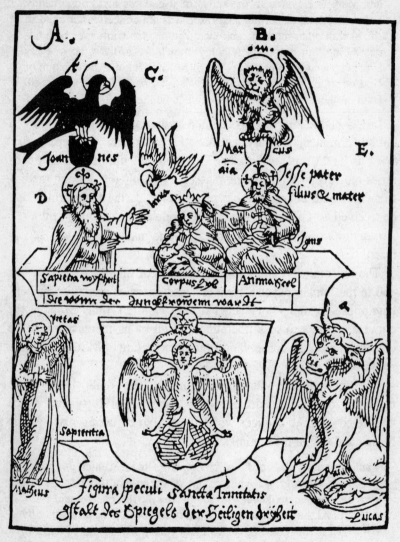

Extraction of Mercurius and coronation of the Virgin.
Lower level: Mercurius being extracted from the *prima materia*.
Upper level: Assumption and coronation of the Virgin.
(*Speculum trinitatis* from Reusner, *Pandora,* 1588)

Then I am outside watching the building. There are two geared wheels connected by a bar attached to the building outside the window of the imprisoned woman. Two small, very agile, acrobats somersault from one wheel to the other, thus turning them. This is very dangerous and we hold our breath but they are highly skilled and manage it safely. The turning of the wheels opens a covering over the large window, revealing the woman who sits in a chair looking out.

I know that when the woman comes down to walk around the square she will come down by a small wooden staircase inside the house.

The dreamer associated the woman at the window with Leonardo da Vinci's *Mona Lisa.* It was in a passage from Marie-Louise von Franz's essay in *Man and His Symbols* that I discovered the key with which to unlock the meaning of this dream. There she speaks of the four-fold structure and development of the feminine archetype, which in a man appears as the anima:

> The first stage is best symbolized by the figure of Eve, which represents purely instinctual and biological relations. The second can be seen in Faust's Helen: She personifies a romantic and aesthetic level that is, however, still characterized by sexual elements. The third is represented, for instance, by the Virgin Mary—a figure who raises love *(eros)* to the heights of spiritual devotion. The fourth type is symbolized by Sapientia, wisdom transcending even the most holy and the most pure. Of this another symbol is the Shulamite in the Song of Solomon. (In the psychic development of modern man this stage is rarely reached. The Mona Lisa comes nearest to such a wisdom anima).[5]

Although von Franz is referring here to the development of a man's anima, the same progression applies to the conscious personality and the Self of a woman. The dream, which combines the third and fourth stages, Mary and the Mona Lisa, suggests that feminine wisdom, long separated from the physical world, living as a captive of the dominant masculine values, is to be lived in a more personal form, once again to walk the surface of the earth, realized in every-

---

[5] "The Process of Individuation," in *Man and His Symbols,* pp. 185-186.

day life. Perhaps the feminine quaternity, which has been split apart, is to be rejoined—body and soul reunited in conscious life.

It would seem that Mary/Mona Lisa/Sophia has been kept in her father's apartment for quite some time. In *The Grail Legend,* Emma Jung and von Franz address at some length the origins of the arrested development of the feminine principle:

> In the medieval *Minnedienst* there was . . . a tendency towards an individual realization of the anima on the one hand, and in the direction of a personal relation to the woman on the other. Because of the increase in the cult of the Virgin, however, both tendencies were cut short. As a result the anima was no longer taken into account, save as an archetypal symbol.[6]

Discussing this situation in a seminar in 1980 at the C.G. Jung Institute in Zurich, von Franz suggested that the cult of the Virgin was fostered in part because of the political and economic problems caused by the large number of bastards, the awkward by-product of concretizing the personal relationships between knights and their lady loves. The prevailing social structure was not yet strong enough to contain the powerful energies of Eros lived in individual earthly form.

Since that time, with feminine development arrested at a collective level, it seems to me that women have by and large been experienced, and have also experienced themselves, more often than not in terms of the collective anima image—the way in which men see women.

Even now it is difficult for an individual woman to make her own way—to find *herself*—in the forest of anima projections which grasp for her ankles like the tangled roots and vines of a primeval forest. A man's unconsciousness of his inner feminine side, coupled with a woman's weak consciousness of herself, weaves an almost impenetrable thicket similar to the one surrounding Sleeping Beauty's castle. The time has come for a path to be opened through the thicket.

---

[6] *The Grail Legend,* p. 155.

Much of the anger of the radical extreme of the women's liberation movement is an attempt, with machetes swinging, to hack a path. But is there not another less destructive way? (The machete, alas, cuts the roses as well as the thorns). A better alternative, it seems to me, is for the individual woman to come to know, if she can, without mercy or self-pity, *who* she is, *what* she is and what is required of her if she is to become more conscious. She must do this in order to know what she is *not,* to differentiate herself from the anima projections which displace her individual expression of the feminine.

Chances are she will not like much of what she will discover—living out a man's anima is, if not more comfortable, at least less strenuous—but if she perseveres she will become more real and responsible for her own life; *Deo concedente,* she will begin to realize her Self.[7]

At the root of a woman's reality lies her physical nature, represented by Helen and Eve, split off from Mary and Sophia. For her male partner the split occurs in the anima, often divided into the opposites of carnal love and idealized beauty. I suggest it is the need to make conscious the chthonic feminine in both men and women, in order to connect it to a reawakened feminine spirit—to reassemble the feminine foursome—which lies beneath the energetic explosion of physical activity in our time.

*

There is a special expression of this renewed interest in the training and use of the body, one in which the opposites of body and spirit have not been completely severed—dance.

Dance, too, has become enormously more popular in recent years. In Boston, for instance, where twenty-five years ago there was one small group of people working in contemporary dance as an art form and perhaps two or three ballet studios, now there are many studios

---

[7] See M. Esther Harding, *The Way of All Women,* especially chap. 1, "All Things to All Men."

teaching contemporary and classical dance, as well as jazz and ballroom. Not just for professional training, these studios cater to a large
amateur clientele. Similarly, the number of performing groups has
greatly increased. Twenty-five years ago an audience of a handful
was considered a good house for an innovative dance company.
Now such groups, as well as traditional ballet companies, can expect
to draw a large audience.

Martha Graham, a great pioneer and genius of contemporary
American dance, developed a new language of the body with which
to sing, with consummate skill and poetry, the images of the soul. In
1960 she choreographed a dance, both witty and poignant, which
she entitled *Acrobats of God.* She took this title from the early
church fathers, "who subjected themselves to the discipline of the
desert . . . the *athletae Dei.*" It was her "fanfare for dance as an art—
a celebration in honor of the trials and tribulations, the discipline, de-
nials, glories and delights of a dancer's world."[8]

Dancers are indeed acrobats of God—or, speaking psychologically, the Self—and the emphasis of their training is on discipline
and denial.

In the dream recounted above, Mary is quiet; the active, moving
energy is embodied in the two acrobats. With their somersaults they
turn the situation around, make visible the Mary/Mona Lisa, hereto-
fore hidden in her father's upstairs apartment—the patterns of the
patriarchy. Somehow these little tumblers seem to aid in bringing her
down to earth, into reality.

We can take these tumblers as animus figures, images of the
dreamer's inner masculine energy and focus. Their duality (the dou-
bling motif in dreams) suggests that a content of the unconscious is
on the brink of becoming conscious.

But also, related as they are to fools and jesters (who were trained
acrobats), the tumblers have a trickster quality. In *The Grail Legend,*

---

[8] Quotations taken from the souvenir program of Martha Graham's 1966
concert season.

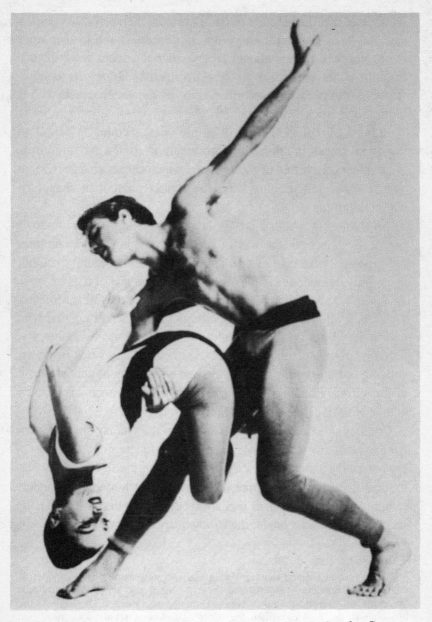

Helen McGehee and Robert Powell in Martha Graham's *Secular Games.*
(Photo by Jack Mitchell)

we are told that the function of the trickster archetype is "to compen-
sate the . . . rigidity in the collective consciousness and to keep open
the approaches to the irrational depths and to the riches of the instinctual and archetypal world."[9] They are ruled by *Mercurius duplex,*
that arch trickster and transformer, spirit of the unconscious, who in
himself combines all opposites.[10]

In fairy tales, a somersault often precedes, seeming to cause, an
important transformation. The somersault, in itself a moving circle,
is a mandala, a symbol of the Self, one which causes change *through
human motion.* Psychologically, this would point to a change of
conscious attitude.

An acrobat may stand on his head, suggesting an upside-down
perspective, an opposite way of seeing things. In this way he joins
the opposites with his physical agility. He is not a natural man, but
one highly trained; discipline of the body, not denial of it, is his way.
And with it he relates to others. He is a servant of the Great Mother.

A medieval story tells of Barnabas, a poor itinerant juggler, who
was invited by a Prior to become a monk and join his monastery.
Finding himself surrounded there by learned and cultivated Brothers,
copying and illustrating manuscripts and composing hymns of praise
to the Virgin, Barnabas fell to lamenting his ignorance, his inability
to give worthy praise to the Mother of God.

One day, when Barnabas was alone in the chapel, the Prior entered in company with two of the oldest Brothers. They saw Barnabas before the statue of the Virgin, his head on the floor and his feet
in the air, juggling six copper balls and twelve knives. Not understanding that the poor man was thus putting his best talents at the
service of Our Lady, one of the Brothers cried out against such sacri-

---

[9] *The Grail Legend,* p. 362.

[10] "I am . . . father and mother, young and old, very strong and very weak,
death and resurrection, visible and invisible, hard and soft; I descend into
the earth and ascend to the heavens, I am the highest and the lowest, the
lightest and the heaviest; often the order of nature is reversed in me . . . I
am dark and light; I come forth from heaven and earth; I am known and yet
do not exist at all . . . . " ("Aurelia occulta," 1659, quoted in Jung, "The
Spirit Mercurius," *Alchemical Studies,* CW 13, par. 267)

lege. All three set about to remove Barnabas from the chapel, when they saw the Virgin slowly descend from the altar and, with a fold of her blue mantle, wipe away the sweat that streamed from the juggler's forehead.

The Prior, bowing his head down to the marble floor, repeated these words: "Blessed are the pure in heart, for they shall see God."[11]

In the dream we are considering, the two acrobats, with their physical energy and skill, can connect Mary/Mona Lisa to everyday reality, revealing her existence and perhaps helping her to descend the wooden staircase to join with those who stand on the ground. She in turn may wipe the sweat from their bodies. The internal wooden staircase suggests this must be done in an introverted, private way, within the individual.

For me, these acrobats, acolytes of the goddess, provide a useful image of the active and creative aspect of a dancer's experience. Like them, through discipline and a kind of asceticism, with sweat and perseverance, dancers shape their bodies, bending them, at least for a time, to the ego's will.

On a personal plane, through fashioning their bodies dancers transform themselves physically and spiritually. Once rooted consciously in the nature of their bodies, dancers become vessels to catch, contain and transform the energies of the unconscious. In their movements they make manifest the images of the transpersonal psyche, bridging the opposites of nature and spirit, earth and sky, everyday life and the infinite.

The training of a dancer parallels in many ways the alchemical *opus,* the psychological significance of which Jung has so perceptively penetrated.[12] By subjecting the initial unformed mass, the *prima materia,* to the operations of heating and dissolving, coagulat-

---

[11] I am indebted to Merle Westlake for this version of Anatole France's tale, *Le Jongleur de Notre Dame.*

[12] See, particularly, *Psychology and Alchemy,* CW 12, *Alchemical Studies,* CW 13 and *Mysterium Coniunctionis,* CW 14.

ing and sublimating, separating and joining, the alchemist endeavored to release the spirit hidden in matter and thus to transform matter itself.[13]

For the alchemist, the glass retort was the vessel of transformation and the matter he labored to transform was outside himself (or so he thought). For anyone undergoing physical training, especially a dancer, both the *prima materia* and the retort are the individual's own body.

Jung discovered that individual psychological transformation—the individuation process—underlay the alchemists' efforts and was projected into the chemical process. For me, physical work, bringing to consciousness at least parts of one's own body, is not only a projection of the individuation process into the body, but also represents a concrete version of the drama. (Indeed, with this in mind I thought of calling this book *The Alchemy of Dance.*)

If this is so, it is only one stage. It is an experience of those archetypal patterns of transformation on the *physical* level. If one is called to pursue one's development psychologically, this physical experience can give the process a dimension which psychological work alone omits: a concrete material dimension, a dimension of the flesh.

Psychological consciousness and understanding is a separate stage of the individuation opus. The dynamism of the instinct lodged in the body must be released to carry on the transformation process in a less concrete way, "through integration of the image which signifies and at the same time evokes the instinct."[14]

Emerson writes that "consciousness in each man is a sliding scale, which identifies him now with the First Cause, and now with the flesh of his body."[15] The psychological quest cannot but be enriched if the realizations and discoveries at the spiritual end of the sliding

---

13 See Edward F. Edinger, *Anatomy of the Psyche: Alchemical Symbolism in Psychotherapy,* for psychological parallels to alchemical operations.

14 "On the Nature of the Psyche," *The Structure and Dynamics of the Psyche,* CW 8, par. 414.

15 Emerson, "Experience," p. 42.

scale are amplified by parallel experiences at the physical end. Expanding consciousness toward matter as well as toward spirit seems to me to be one way of reuniting Eve and Helen with Mary and Sophia—concrete matter and instinct with feminine love and wisdom.

Having myself been both victim and beneficiary of the physical compulsion to train my body, to relate it to consciousness in order that I might be a dancer, an acrobat of the gods, I have over the past twenty years been reflecting on the meaning of that effort.

What is dance? What is physical consciousness and how is it achieved? What is the purpose of making the body a responsive instrument of the ego and a servant of the spirit? What is the secret, the value, contained in the body, in physical activity, in matter, and how can it be extracted from the *massa confusa* of the unconscious?

Some possible answers to these questions are the substance of this book.

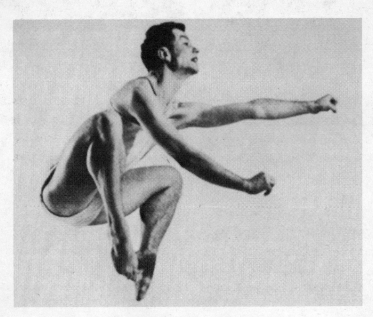

Merce Cunningham.
(Photo by Gerda Peterich)

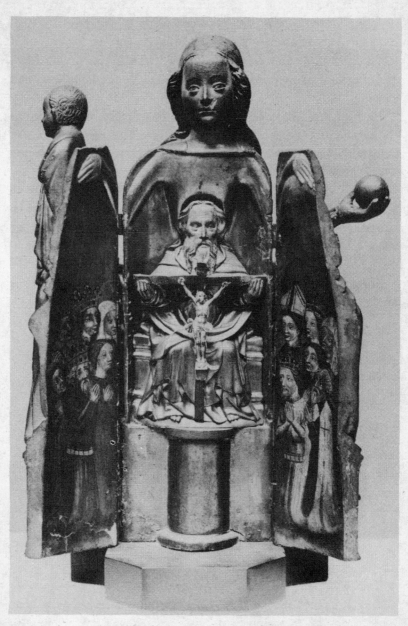

The Virgin Mary as vessel.
(Painted wood, France, 15th cent.)

2
The Vessel

> For this task [reconciliation of the opposites] the individual human being serves as a *vessel*, for only when the opposites are reconciled in the single individual can they be united. The individual therefore becomes a receptacle for the transformation of the problem of the opposites in the image of God. . . . Each human being represents a place of transformation and a "vessel" in which God may come to consciousness.
> —Emma Jung and Marie-Louise von Franz, *The Grail Legend.*

It is the tension between a myriad of opposites which creates both the dance and the dancer. Dancing springs into life because of the interplay of many opposing forces—within the body itself, between the body and psyche of the dancer, and between the dancer, the audience and the surrounding forces of time and space. In this chapter I will examine some of these polarities and try to separate the coils of clay with which the vessel is formed.

The Sacred in Dance

First and foremost we encounter the opposites of the profane and the sacred. Anyone who enters the realm of danced theater enters even now, when dance seems so secular, a sacred realm. Behind the effort needed to become a dancer, as I see it, lies a deep urge to be allowed into sacred time and space, to open the earthly body and what it can communicate to an other-worldly energy.

The dance itself becomes, for a moment, the vessel into which sacred energies may flow, a vehicle for the manifestation of the gods, those forces which appear in the psyche as archetypal images. No experience is as fully alive as having that god-like energy move

23

through one. A priest, a shaman, a lover, a performer, and yes, sometimes even an analyst, knows and longs for that heightened sense of life and purpose. The wise know enough to say, "Not I, but the god in me," or, "It used me."

The danger of identification with the transcendent energy is always present, and it is ever needful to guard against thinking "I" did it. Primitive dancers become possessed and perform superhuman feats in a state of ecstasy, their nascent egos totally eclipsed. A dancer whose training makes the body a partially conscious instrument, to some extent under the aegis of the ego, is still reaching for a piece of that ecstasy—not consciously, perhaps, but nonetheless, as she or he strives for perfect line, elevation, control, rhythm, design, expression, the goal is to embody an archetypal image for others.

Alas, this goal is all too often contaminated with the concupiscent ego's lust for fame. There is always a danger that the performer will identify with the archetypal image he or she represents. How often, even now, I still experience some of this sin of inflation when I say (now suspicious of the prideful note in my voice), "I used to be a dancer"—hoping, fishing, for a response of wonder from my audience.

An acquaintance of mine who was a friend of two famous dancers once described an important difference he noticed between them. One was always himself, on stage and off. A great dancer, yes, but he and his role were identical. He was inflated by his identification with the gods. The other one did not succumb to this inflation. After a performance it would sometimes take him an hour or so before he could even speak; he was, as it were, still absent, so completely had he been at the service of the role he had been dancing. You had the feeling that his ego was not identified with his role but rather its servant. Like a shaman, he was a vehicle through which the divine could flow.

Costumes, masks and theater make-up are psychologically of great value for the performer in guarding against inflation. The rituals of donning the mask, the persona, and of shedding it at the end of the performance, mark for the wary the boundary between the oppo-

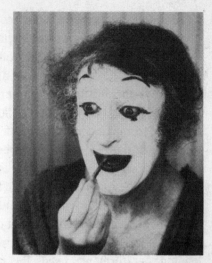

Marcel Marceau.
(Photo by Ben Martin)

site realms of the personal and the archetypal, the ego and the Self. At the end of the performance one sheds the god's shape—unless, that is, one has had the misfortune to become glued to it.

The stage, the altar, the dance studio, are sacred spaces, and the dancing time, the learning time, is time out of our time. Each class is a physical meditation. One ballet teacher crosses herself before starting each class, and everyone finishes with a *reverence;* first a bow to her own ballet master's photograph and then a bow to the crucifix in the opposite corner of the studio. These can be called "nothing but" gestures, yet often both student and teacher feel a numinous surge at the ritual.

Another teacher I knew used to make a special point of sending her students out of the studio and then asking them to return, *consciously,* sensing the difference between the busy hallway outside and the quiet studio space. For her, the studio was hallowed—a *temenos,* the goddess's sacred ground, dedicated to and ruled by forces which were not personal.[1]

---

[1] The analyst's consulting room can have a similar quality. The *temenos* was originally a sacred precinct, often dedicated to the goddess Gaia. See Jung, *Symbols of Transformation,* CW 5, par. 570.

After one enters the sacred space there is, ideally, a period of quieting down. Many classes start with slow breathing. Physiologically, the warming and tuning of the body must proceed slowly to avoid injury. But psychologically, too, after the hassle of rushing to the studio and the bustle and chatter of the dressing room, quiet is needed to bring one's scattered thoughts to a still, introverted point of focus, to make connection with the other world. "Except for the point, the still point, there would be no dance, and there is only the dance."[2]

So also, the *rites d'entrée* before a performance: the careful warm-up of the body, the costuming and donning of the mask of make-up—and often dancers meditate or do yoga before performing. All of this is not unrelated to the prayer upon entering a church. For me, attending a performance needs the same ritual: getting to the theater early enough not to feel rushed, entering the sacred space consciously, being quiet for a moment—to be part of the call to the gods to come down amongst the mortal audience and performers.

Ritual permeates the world of the dancer, whether student or performer, amateur or professional. With it, like the bucket sent down into a well, the water of life is reached and drawn up into the conscious realm. Yes, the dancing ground is a sacred eternal space, the dancing time also, and one is calling to the gods to enter one's body and being.

Yet, if the dancing space and dancing time are other-worldly, there is nothing out of this world about the matter of the dancer—his or her body. Everything is the matter! This stuff, these bones, "this too, too solid flesh,"[3] are truly down to earth and mundane, quite the opposite of the sacred space in time in which the dancer, trained or untrained, will move. Here the polarities of this and the other world mingle, indeed are muddled.

I still remember vividly, when I was one of a class of rank beginners, being told by the teacher never to expect any help whatsoever

---

2 T.S. Eliot, "Burnt Norton," lines 66-67.
3 William Shakespeare, *Hamlet,* act 1, scene 2.

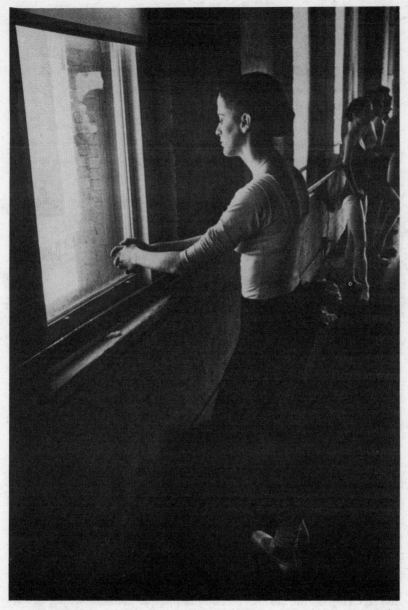

"Quiet is needed to bring one's scattered thoughts to a still, introverted
point of focus, to make connection with the other world."
(Photo by Earl Dotter)

from our bodies. The body, appallingly subject to the pull of gravity—the Great Goddess at her most insistent—longs to sit still, to
sink into its mother soil. It reacts with pain, lethargy, obstinacy to
the efforts of the dancer to move and train it. From the very start of
dance training one is torn between the opposites of the body's lethargy and the ego's will.

Before examining this separation, the conflict which potentially
leads to differentiation and consciousness, let us look for a moment
at the original unity of body and ego, the *prima materia* of the vessel.

Ego-Body Identity

> There is, in the first place, a certain identity with the body. . . .
> [This] is one of the first things which makes an ego; it is the spatial
> separateness that induces, apparently, the concept of an ego.[4]

In the beginning we are identical with our bodies, and each body
bears the unmistakable stamp of the human animal—the anatomical
organization is the same for each individual. Yet, although in so
many ways we are alike, we all look different. I remember my surprise when as a child I learned that no two fingerprints were the
same, and, much later, the sense of wonder when I saw the foot-
prints of my first child, the unique expression of a universal pattern.

From birth, the opposites of individual and collective are present,
anchored, portrayed in each human body. In the beginning, individual and collective, body and psyche, are one. Out of this original
wholeness emerges the differentiated individual. The goal toward
which we are thrust is a second wholeness—wholeness which ideally results, at the end of life, from the weaving together of threads
separated during the effort to become conscious.

Reality begins with the body, which gives us shape, existence and
boundaries. It is the carrier of our being in the world, the *sine qua
non* of living on the earth. The body is the one element which distin-

---

4 Jung, quoted in Richard I. Evans, *Conversations with Carl Jung,* p. 41.

guishes this life from any existence the soul or psyche might have in other worlds.

As far as we know, only within a body is human growth, psychological and physical, possible. It is our ark, our whale, the ego's womb. It can also be our teacher, leading us to discover what is not possible, bounding us to the utmost.[5] The awareness that "I" am this body, "I" am finite and separate from other bodies, forms the skeleton of the ego.

Of late I have become increasingly conscious of the importance of *touch,* of tactile awareness both within the body and between the body and the outer environment—that sense of "spatial separateness" which seems to be necessary for the definition of the ego.

A study aired on television in 1980 investigated the importance of touch in the development of humans and other animals. Baby chimpanzees who were separated by a sheet of glass from their mothers and thus denied tactile contact with them, were found to have suffered severe brain damage. This was not so for the control group, which had full tactile contact with their mothers.[6] These experiments suggest that an individual's connection to the world, the awareness of oneself, is dependent on touching and being touched.[7]

The absence of tactile sensation seems to melt the boundaries between ego and unconscious. John Lilly, a physicist who has experimented with altered states of consciousness, reports that one way to induce an hallucinatory state is to float for a period of time in an isolation tank. In this environment external tactile sensations are almost entirely eliminated.[8]

With this in mind—and looking at it upside-down, like an acrobat—it has occurred to me that the difficulty many people experience

---

[5] See Jung, *Memories, Dreams, Reflections,* p. 324.

[6] Stephen Rose, producer, "A Touch of Sensitivity," pp. 8-9.

[7] This subject is explored in Deldon Anne McNeely, *Touching: Body Therapy and Depth Psychology,* esp. pp. 62ff.

[8] See *The Center of the Cyclone,* esp. pp. 38ff. An isolation tank is a container of water at body temperature, in a darkened and silent room, in which the subject floats for varying periods of time.

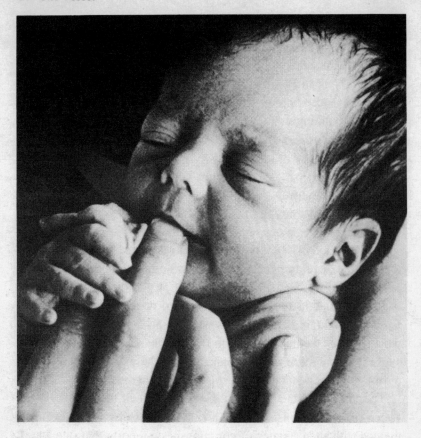

in doing what Jung called active imagination may stem from an *over-awareness* of the body.[9] Perhaps a too highly developed sensory awareness inhibits fantasy. If too little awareness of the body sweeps us off our feet, does too much keep us stuck to the ground?

It is in psychotic states, particularly schizophrenia, that we see how the absence of tactile definition—the lack of physical bound-

---

[9] Active imagination is a process by which one interacts consciously with contents of the unconscious. This may take many forms, including drawing or painting, writing, sculpting or dance. See Jung, "The Transcendent Function," *The Structure and Dynamics of the Psyche,* CW 8, pars. 166-175, and Barbara Hannah, *Encounters with the Soul: Active Imagination as Developed by C.G. Jung.*

aries—can cause serious trouble. An ego not anchored in the reality of the body is fragile, susceptible to being swamped by the unconscious. The injuries schizophrenics inflict on themselves—cigarette burns, wrist slashing, sticking their feet into fire, head knocking, for example—may be attempts to awaken some sensation, a sense of life, into an otherwise numb body.[10]

A chronic schizophrenic, well aware of her needs, once asked me to work with her in movement. Not understanding the depth of her physical deprivation, I started at too advanced a level, suggesting she move her fingers to become more aware of them. She later told me she had been so confused that she had to withdraw into a catatonic state. The process was too complicated for her. Subsequently, with her therapist, it was regression to the state of infancy, being held closely as a babe, which took her to the place where healing could begin.

The Body as Shadow

> For the body is a terribly awkward thing and so it is omitted; we can deal with things spiritually so much more easily without the despicable body.[11]

The body and its sense of touch is very important for the development of the ego. Yet in order to develop the spirit and rational consciousness, Christianity had historically to declare the body untouchable—a kind of second-class citizen. The price many of us must pay for this is that the body becomes a problem.

Untouched, repressed, denied, the body moves into the shadow, where dwell those aspects of ourselves we are loath to look at. Then the ego loses a direct connection to the body as a source of natural wisdom and energy. Jung writes:

---

[10] A healing approach to the absence of body awareness is illustrated in the case of Renée, recounted in Marguerite Sechehaye, *Autobiography of a Schizophrenic Girl,* esp. pp. 73, 112. There the growth of a "body ego" is fostered by a great deal of tactile contact, such as holding and bathing.

[11] Jung, *Nietzsche's Zarathustra,* p. 63.

We do not like to look at the shadow-side of ourselves; therefore there are many people in our civilized society who have lost their shadow altogether, they have got rid of it. They are only two-dimensional; they have lost the third dimension, and with it they have usually lost the body. The body is a most doubtful friend because it produces things we do not like; there are too many things about the body which cannot be mentioned. The body is very often the personification of this shadow of the ego. Sometimes it forms the skeleton in the cupboard, and everybody naturally wants to get rid of such a thing.[12]

Any "skeleton in the cupboard" behaves like an autonomous complex. Its vitality remains undiminished but instead of being a contributing partner to consciousness, the body goes its isolated way, creating compulsions, eating disorders, injuries, physical illnesses and of course many psychological problems.

Denied the attention and care it merits, the body presses its demand for attention in a hostile, destructive way. This is "the body's revenge upon the spirit."[13] It is to bring a stop to the war between the opposites of body and spirit, nature and culture, that nature, the unconscious, now involves so many of us in "a re-estimation of the basic facts of human nature,"[14] a renewed interest in relating to the positive aspects of our own bodies.

Just as the first step in the individuation process is the recognition of the personal shadow and its integration back into the ego complex, so too the renewed interest in physical activity of all sorts serves to reconnect once again shadowed *physis* with psyche.

Why Dance?

Let us return to the world of the dancer. Over the years I have continually asked myself why people start to dance. Many are simply born dancers—a high level of kinesthetic and creative energy decrees

---

12 "The Tavistock Lectures," *The Symbolic Life,* CW 18, par. 40.
13 Jung. *Modern Man in Search of a Soul,* p. 219.
14 Ibid.

that their's is to be a dancer's life. At the same time, they often have a troubled relationship with their bodies.

Violette Verdy, the great French-American ballerina, gives the following description of her path to dance:

> I had a very delicate liver as a kid. If it wasn't watched carefully, I could be slowly poisoned and go into a coma. My mother took me to a famous pediatrician, who prescribed a diet that we followed very carefully, and I began to grow stronger. And then my mother complained that I was almost hyperactive—I wouldn't eat, wouldn't sleep, and was always restless. The doctor said, "Well, we will have to tire her out. But it would be nice to tire her out in a harmonious way, so why don't you have her study some sort of dancing?" And my mother said that although she had never seen ballet except for pictures, she had a tremendous admiration for its structure and discipline. And she had an idea that there was something in the way I behaved that indicated a spirit that should be considered. And it was a good thing, because to become a ballet dancer you have to decide so early. So we moved to Paris when I was eight.[15]

Most dancers I have known, amateur or professional, started during or after adolescence because in one way or another their bodies were for them "a terribly awkward thing." One man sought to heal a wound incurred in the Second World War, another to overcome the effects of polio; still another came to dance because of recurring boils and muscular weakness.

Some (especially women) are drawn to dance because of a feeling of being fat and ungraceful, and others because of a vague longing for something more vital in their lives. Many dancers have a need, conscious or instinctive, to reconnect with, or better utilize, the life force inherent in the body. It is safe to say that somewhere in the picture there is usually a reflection of the shadowed, disturbed state of Mother Nature herself.

A group of us, in an adult beginner's class, were sitting around discussing why such poor physical specimens as ourselves—disjointed, ungainly, fat, unhappy with our bodies—were driven to

---

[15] Cynthia Lyle, *Dancers on Dancing*, p. 62.

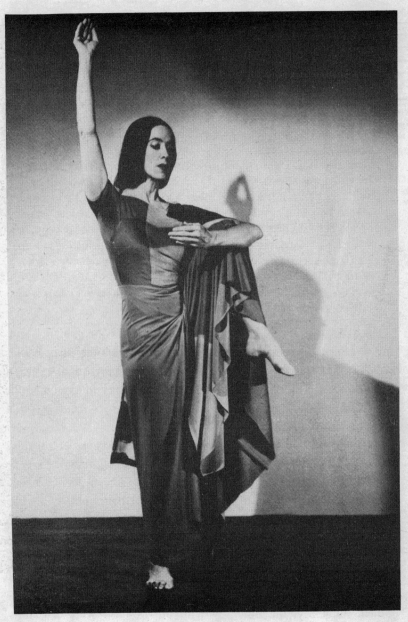

Martha Graham in *Indian Episode*.
(Photo by Barbara Morgan)

dance. Our teacher's answer remains vivid in my memory: "It is one of the few ways you can tangibly work on yourselves, improve yourselves. Only those who need the work are driven to it."

The urge to work on the body seems often to come from an instinct to heal a split or injury, a malformation or deadness within, and, importantly, to strengthen the ego as well as the body, by awakening the body to consciousness. It is a version of work on the physical side of both the personal and collective aspects of the shadow—a form of regression, perhaps, but only so in the sense characterized by Jung as "a *reculer pour mieux sauter* [a step back, the better to leap ahead], an amassing and integration of powers that will develop into a new order."[16]

For many, then, dance is an effort at healing, but one which, as Violette Verdy's mother sensed, includes the spirit as well as the body.

Although many of the physiological aspects of training apply equally to classical ballet, my focus here, by and large, is with modern dancers, men and women who have followed the lead of the great innovators of the twentieth century: Isadora Duncan, Ruth St. Denis, Mary Wigman, Martha Graham, to name only the most important. These pioneers broke with the rigid constraints of classical dance to build a new art form; searching for ways to express contemporary experience, they created a new movement vocabulary.

Ballet was born in the court of Louis XIV and was shaped thereafter almost exclusively by male choreographers; the female dancer, *en pointe,* touching the earth like a feather, reflects the feminine image of a man's soul—the anima. The people who broke away from the classical forms at the start of the twentieth century and rejuvenated the art of dance were, importantly, women. It was Isadora Duncan who, at the turn of the century, dared to free the body. She stripped off corset and point shoes and, copying the ancient Greeks, danced in her bare feet wearing only a thin silk tunic and scarves.

---

[16] "Principles of Practical Psychotherapy," *The Practice of Psychotherapy,* CW 16, par. 19.

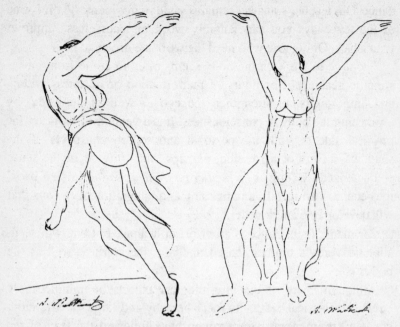

Isadora Duncan, by Abraham Walkowitz.

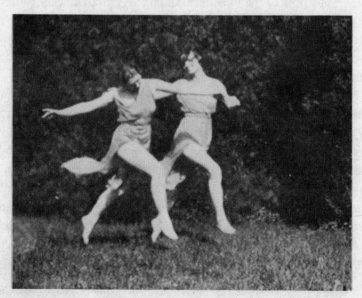

Duncan dancers in the 1930s.

The new dance was a search for more natural movement. In 1905, Duncan wrote:

> The true dance is appropriate to the most beautiful human form; the false dance is the opposite of this definition—that is, that movement which conforms to a deformed human body. First, draw me the form of a woman as it is in Nature, and now draw me the form of a woman in a . . . corset and the satin slippers used by . . . [ballet] dancers. To the first all the rhythmic movements that run through Nature would be possible. . . . To the second figure these movements would be impossible on account of the rhythm being broken and stopped at the extremities.[17]

Modern dancers, their bodies freed to move in countless new ways, turn to the floor —to the earth —as adversary, for support, as a partner. Whilst a ballerina strives to create an illusion of weightlessness and often is held aloft beyond the pull of gravity by her partner, modern dancers, men and women alike, do not shun gravity's insistence. Instead of trying to escape the floor, they lie on it, kneel, turn and twist on it, fall to it and rise from it. Consciously in touch with the earth, their movements communicate that earthen reality. Acrobats of the gods and goddesses, they bring Mary down to earth from the prison of her father's apartment.

For the woman who is a modern dancer, the informing archetype is still the Kore, the Greek maiden goddess;[18] no dancer wants to be fat or matronly. But she is a Kore born of Demeter, the Earth Goddess—not, as in classical ballet, born of the idealized image of woman in a masculine mind's eye.

If many individual dancers turn to the rigors of dance training to heal some malaise within themselves, I think it can also be said that the emergence of the new form of dance is an expression of an im-

---

17 Quoted in Elizabeth Kendall, *Where She Danced,* p. 60. This book is especially valuable for its account of the emergence of modern dance as an aspect of the contemporary ground-swell to free the female body—a manifestation of the evolution of the feminine archetype at the start of the twentieth century.

18 See Jung, "The Psychological Aspects of the Kore," *The Archetypes and the Collective Unconscious,* CW 9i, pars. 306, 311.

pulse in the collective unconscious to heal the split in the feminine archetype and to stop the war between Mother Earth and Father Sky.

In this sense both the dancer and the dance become, as suggested in the passage at the head of this chapter, "a receptacle for the transformation of the problem of the opposites."

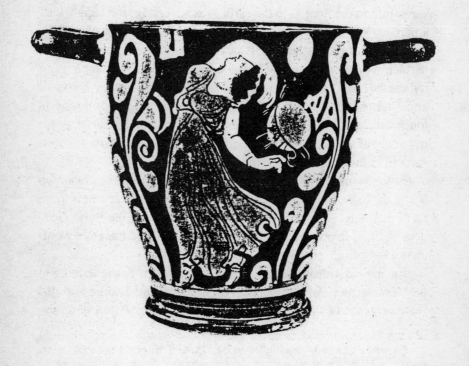

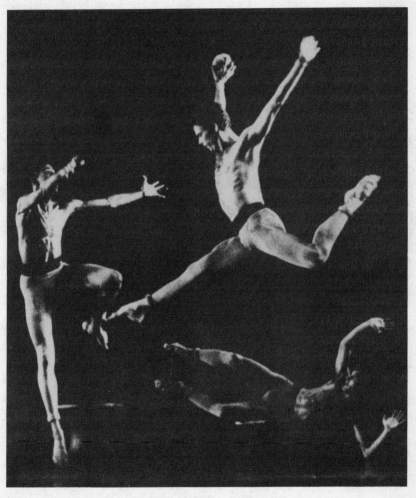
Robert Powell and the Graham Company in *Secular Games.*
(Photo by Martha Swope)

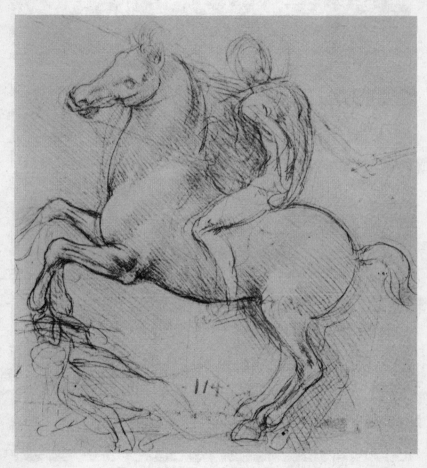

Horse and Rider, by Leonardo da Vinci.

3
Preparing the Body

Without realizing the animal that is within you, how could
you ever understand yourself? . . . You can only know yourself
if you really get into yourself, and you can only do that if you
accept the lead of the animal.
—C.G. Jung, *The Visions Seminars.*

Regression carried to its logical conclusion means a linking
back with the world of natural instincts, which in its formal or
ideal aspect is a kind of *prima materia.* If this *prima materia*
can be assimilated by the conscious mind it will bring about a
reactivation and reorganization of its contents.
—C.G. Jung, *Symbols of Transformation.*

The Process

People who are driven to do something about their bodies are led
back to the world of nature. A dancer's training is an investigation, a
venture into one's animal ancestry, a discovery of the anatomy and
character of one's own horse. One returns to the realm of the physical aspect of instincts, and to their chthonic energy.

In his *Visions Seminars,* Jung speaks of "regression to the
Dionysian point of view, through contact with the earth."[1] Dance is
indeed such a regression. But dance training is a slow process of rediscovery, so that consciousness is not obliterated in a frenzy of possession; instead it does the leading, the dismembering, the investigat-
ing; it contains and controls.

The rider who gets to know the horse also learns from it. The
mind is always there, observing, connecting, listening, pushing,

---

[1] *The Visions Seminars,* vol. 1, p. 164.

eventually learning to respect the limitations of the physical instrument as well as encouraging it to perform beyond its natural capacity.

In the psychological realm it is the instinctual drives such as sexuality, hunger, power, which must be explored in the painful light of the investigator's lantern—instincts which have been put in the shadow by Western efforts to become civilized and rational. Released, explored and redirected, these energies can greatly enrich life.

So too, in training the body to dance, the natural energy inherent in muscles and blood, the instinctive pulse of rhythm, is harnessed to a potentially creative process and redirected for spiritual growth.

The analytic process stretches consciousness toward the psychological end of the matter-psyche spectrum, promoting an awareness and understanding of image, an appreciation of life on a symbolic level.[2] Physical work stretches the field of consciousness in the opposite direction, toward a greater connection with the material end of the spectrum. When the individual can relate to both, one pole informs the other.

The Third Eye

> According to [a] Yakut account, the evil spirits carry the future shaman's soul to the underworld and there shut it up in a house for three years .... Here the shaman undergoes his initiation. The spirits cut off his head, which they set aside (for the candidate must watch his dismemberment with his own eyes), and cut him into small pieces which are then distributed to the spirits of the various diseases. Only by undergoing such an ordeal will the future shaman gain the power to cure. His bones are then covered with new flesh, and in some cases he is also given new blood.[3]

The training of a dancer is not unlike the initiation of a shaman, though it often takes *ten* years in the underworld space of the dance

---

[2] "Man is in need of a symbolic life .... Where do we live symbolically? Nowhere, except where we participate in the ritual of life. But who, among the many, are really participating in the ritual of life? Very few." (Jung, "The Symbolic Life," *The Symbolic Life,* CW 18, par. 625.

[3] Mircea Eliade, *Shamanism: Archaic Techniques of Ecstasy,* pp. 36-37.

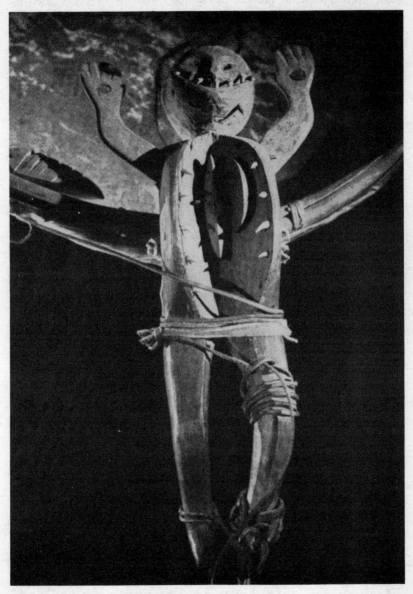
Dancing spirit on shaman's drum.
(Photo by Eberhard Otto)

studio to complete the process of the body's dismemberment and renewal. Certainly, and above all, "the candidate must watch his dismemberment with his own eyes."

It is this watching, this constantly focused attention, which enlarges consciousness and differentiates the training process from Dionysian possession. From the start, the development of a third eye, objectivity, is central to the process. This gradually leads to a separation of the doer from the doing, the ego from the body.

The teacher is of course the student's first experience of the observing eye. When body and ego are still identical, the observing function is projected outside, indeed can only come from there. It is the teacher who points out that one's belly is hanging out, the pelvis not correctly held, that the right knee turns in over the foot, or that one is using the left instead of the right arm in an exercise, and very probably the wrong muscle with which to lift it.

The teacher sets the exercise, the tempo, the rhythm and then constantly corrects the execution. The teacher is the other, the leader, in effect the analyst.

It is no surprise that a strong transference often develops in this situation, an experience I had to the hilt with my first teacher. He provided a good hook for the projection: a glorious dancer, a fine teacher, a wise man. But it was not until I, as a teacher myself, experienced exaggerated admiration from my students—and knew full well that it was out of line with my own reality—that I began to sense that something was at work in the psychological realm. An energy was present that had little to do with my personal merits as a teacher. That was, in fact, one of the puzzles which aroused my curiosity and led me from dance to psychology.

The second tool which is essential to the development of objectivity is the mirror, that ubiquitous reflecting presence in every dance studio. Like Narcissus gazing into the pool, a would-be dancer spends a great deal of time watching his or her reflection.

Learning to use the mirror correctly, however, is a task in itself, for one can, again like Narcissus, become stuck to it and lose touch with the physical sensations within the body, with reality. In addi-

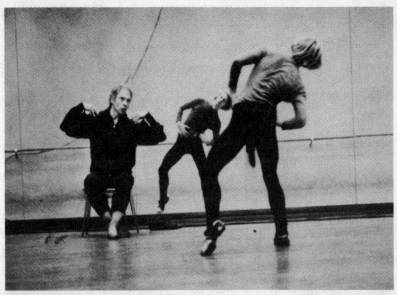

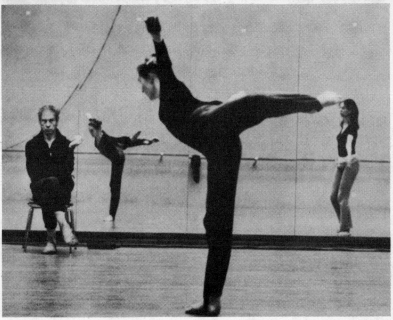

"The teacher is the student's first experience of the observing eye."
(Merce Cunningham in rehearsal; photos by James Klosty)

tion, especially at the start, the image one encounters in the mirror is usually so discouraging that the student is tempted to ignore the reflection of his or her imperfections and remain instead in the fantasy world of illusion. The ideal to which one aspires is far pleasanter than the hulking sight of the untrained, unsculpted body.

This is of course an encounter with the shadow. Learning to face it takes as much courage on the physical level as it does on the psychological level, and when one faces it, one learns a lesson in objectivity.[4]

The mirror is a merciless critic, as Snow White's stepmother discovered to her fury. Occasionally, there is that wonderful moment when one checks in the mirror and sees with some astonishment a creature who actually looks like a dancer. The mirror is an invaluable tool for seeing both one's imperfections and one's progress. That image in the mirror is the dancer; now that I can see what she looks like, I can help her to improve. She and I are sisters, perhaps, but no longer identical.

There are dangers, however. I have seen a neurotic dancer experience herself entirely in the mirror image, losing all sense of herself as the object outside the looking glass. Projecting herself completely into the mirror, she ceased to exist without it. This is a split rather than a differentiation, akin to an out-of-body experience; it is depersonalization.

To counteract the inadequacies and very real dangers of such a one-sided, extraverted orientation, it is extremely important to develop inner sensations—an inner sense of touch—sources of information about what is really happening as one dances.

I taught in one dance studio where we were fortunate enough to have curtains which could be drawn across the wall of mirrors at the front of the studio. When one works without the mirror—and sometimes I would have my students work with their eyes closed to further intensify the experience—one becomes aware of that most im-

---

[4] See Marion Woodman, *Addiction to Perfection*, pp. 99-101, for a discussion of a daily journal as "silver mirror" in psychological work.

portant sixth sense: *proprioceptivity,* the kinesthetic sense within the body. Located in the muscles, joints and tendons, the kinesthetic sense tells the ego from within what is happening—the shape of a movement, whether a foot is correctly pointed, a knee cap held taut, the spine stretched, the head balanced properly, the shoulders easy.

The correct use of the mirror involves a shifting of the focus from outer perception to inner, a constant back and forth between sensing what a movement feels like from within and seeing what it looks like from outside. Gradually one develops an ability to be in two places at once: on the stage, performing, and in the audience, watching.

Dance as a performing art stresses an extraverted mode—one moves for the teacher, the mirror, other students and ultimately for an audience. But good training and good performing must develop and use the inner eye as well. Just as in psychological training one gradually learns to depend on one's inner experience of reality— withdrawing projections from the external world and acquiring some independence of the analyst—so too the dancer, no longer relying solely on a reflected image for knowledge of the body's shape and movement, becomes his or her own observer.

The following passage describes how Doris Humphrey, a superb dancer and choreographer, experienced the third eye. It is also a good example of a dancer's use of active imagination.

> Every moment now is consumed in making every move in my dances as finished as possible—or in thinking about them. Early in the morning I begin seeing a figure, myself, dancing on a stage, and I, the onlooker, am always above and at a distance from it. Quite often, as it is going through the sequence of a dance, it will do a new gesture, and if this pleases the onlooker, the figure will do it over and over, quite obligingly, in fact with considerable satisfaction. But this is a tiring process, my bones ache and I want the dancer to let me rest. But she won't. She fades into a mist temporarily, and then begins again on some other dance, quite amazingly bright and strong. And this goes on all day—day after day on subways, on buses, anywhere, an absolute slavery.[5]

5 Selma Jeanne Cohen, ed., *Doris Humphrey: An Artist First,* p. 107.

Earlier, I suggested that the body, and with it the ego, may find and secure its boundaries by being touched externally. This plants the individual in reality. Feeling the body from within, proprioceptively, has a similar value, with the added benefit that the individual does not rely exclusively on outer stimulation but touches, feels, oneself. This process is akin to withdrawing projections in psychological development. Shadow/body and ego once again speak to each other and enter into an active experience of the wholeness of the organism in which they both play such an important part. This is perhaps why physical activity generally makes us feel better—it heals the separation (or out-and-out split) between body and non-body.

It may be that external contact has to come first, initiating the original sense of differentiation between mother and child, the birth of the separate ego. Eventually, however, at least for those for whom the body presents a problem, the quest for wholeness is furthered by the conscious realization of the inner tactile sense.

The dawning of the inner sensation function, the kinesthetic sense, comes when consciousness turns its attention to physical experiences within the body.

The Sixth Sense

Those wishing to become trained dancers begin with little or no ability to control their bodies, beyond what is instinctively acquired. They cannot really feel themselves, they do not yet possess their bodies or their physiological centers.

The situation is similar to one Barbara Hannah describes:

> Balance in bicycling is an instinctive matter; once we have learned to ride a bicycle we do so quite unconsciously. If, however, we begin to think about where we should place our weight, the chances are that we will lose our instinctive balance at once. It could be done, no doubt, by a careful and long synchronization of balance and thought, but very few people would be willing to make the effort.[6]

---

[6] *Striving Towards Wholeness,* p. 3

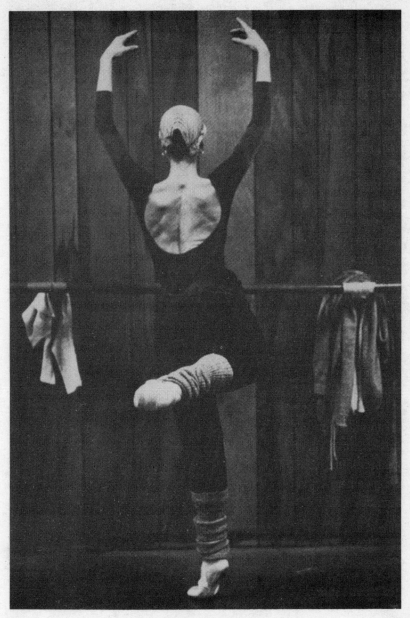

Feeling the body from within, proprioceptively.
(Photo by Earl Dotter)

A dancer is one of those few people who is willing to, and indeed for one reason or another must, make that effort. But it is true—the instinctive coherence, the preconscious totality, collapses as soon as one tries to make the process conscious.

A simple movement, such as walking down the street with arms and legs swinging in opposition (the left arm swings forward with the right leg), is completely natural when one doesn't think about it. For most beginners, however, when a teacher asks them to do this consciously, it becomes an almost impossible task. I have seen well-coordinated athletes fall apart when they try to walk in this simple, "natural" way.

Interestingly, they regress to a more archaic movement pattern, one which comes from a very early stage of neurological development. Rather than moving the arms and legs in opposition, they move one side of the body, arm and leg together, and then the other. When asked to do this consciously, they quickly feel how awkward it is.[7]

This parallels the shaman's dismemberment: the beginner feels like a pile of separated, unconnected bones lying in a jumbled heap. The training process must start from this initial chaos to sort out and reconnect the dismembered parts, put new muscles on the bones, new blood (feeling) into the body. It is like developing a telephone or radio network between hitherto isolated communities and a central government.

The building of this neurological telephone network requires the awakening of a sixth sense. Although common parlance understands a sixth sense as an intuitive hunch ("a power of perception seemingly independent of the five senses"),[8] those concerned with training the body know there is a different sixth sense, one which is absolutely essential for a dancer. This is the kinesthetic sense and it is no less sensory a source of physical information than tasting, smelling,

---

[7] Martha Graham has intentionally incorporated this archaic mode into her movement vocabulary.

[8] Definition in *American Heritage Dictionary*.

touching, seeing and hearing. It is in fact a tactile sense, located not on the skin's surface but within the muscles, tendons and joints.

Raoul Gelabert describes the kinesthetic sense as follows:

> This is . . . known as "position sense," for it is the sense that gives the awareness of the position of the parts of the body without the aid of vision or touch.
>
> There are three types of receptors, which are sense organs in the nerve endings, that record muscle sensations. One of these is located in the fleshy part of the muscle, another in the tendons close to the point of union with the muscle proper, and the third in the fasciae [a sheet of fibrous tissue beneath the surface of the skin] of the muscles. These receptors are responsible for making us aware of the state that a muscle is in—whether it's contracted or stretched, as well as the intensity of the contraction or stretch. . . .
>
> The kinesthetic sense enables us to know with a fair degree of accuracy, the position of any part of the body and the movement that a part of the body is undergoing even when that part is moved by someone else.[9]

This inner sensing is developed first through a constant repetition of exercises; in combination with correct breathing (extremely important), the muscles, tendons and joints are used over and over again. At the start it is the teacher who is responsible for overseeing this. His or her watching and knowledge of correct placement and movement are essential. In training the preadolescent dancers in Bali, in fact, the dancer herself remains completely passive, as in a trance, while the master stands behind, manipulating her limbs in the correct shape and rhythm, programming her as it were.

Through constant repetition, as the muscles gain in strength and memory, the inner sense develops. The combination of constantly increasing usage, of patterning and correction from without, the dancer's checking in the mirror and focusing on the sensations inside the body, all contribute to a specific kinesthetic knowledge of what is happening in the body.

---

[9] William Como, *Raoul Gelabert's Anatomy for the Dancer*, vol. 1, pp. 32-33.

Gradually, as one learns what correct placement and movement feel like, one can correct oneself, no longer dependent on being read from outside. The ego becomes conscious of what "I" am doing and what "I" look like.

For the most part, early training takes place in a collective situation, in the dance studio, but as the kinesthetic sense grows, there develops for many dancers a conflict between working in a class, where one is told what to do and how to do it, and working alone, where one can listen more closely to one's own body. Introversion and extraversion collide.

I first experienced this when, after I had reached a certain degree of proficiency, I began to have strong resistances to going into the city to take class. Whereas earlier I had flown in eagerly, I began to find all manner of complications in the outer world to block my way: the late afternoon traffic became too much to fight, I couldn't find baby sitters to take care of my children, I was too tired, etc., etc. This conflict had various components, but in retrospect I think the central one was the conflict between collective and individual ways of working and experiencing myself.

It was when I was teaching that I began to understand the problem. If I told the class to stretch a certain muscle, I could see that for at least some of my students it was the wrong command. For a person with a certain configuration of the knee, for instance, stretching was not what was needed but rather a special kind of contraction of the muscles which holds the knee-cap taut. Yet with twenty students and a limited amount of time, I could not hope to tailor my commands to each unique body. I was forced to give a general instruction which would work more or less for most of the students, but not suit anyone exactly.[10]

If, as a student, I forced myself to go to a group class, I too would be compelled to conform to a pattern which often differed

---

[10] This problem is of course not specific to training dancers; it is the unavoidable consequence of dealing with statistical averages in any walk of life. As Jung points out, "Statistics obliterate everything unique." *(Mysterium Coniunctionis,* CW 14, par. 194)

from my own physical peculiarities or my needs for that day. On the other hand, when I worked out by myself, although I could enter my inner landscape with far greater concentration, I found it much harder to whip myself up to the level of energy which could be generated when working in a class. I couldn't make myself jump as high or as often, run as much, execute turns as difficult (especially to the left!). I would get sloppy and could not watch for my own mistakes with the same eagle eye as my teacher.

Both ways have value. The collective, extraverted class pushes one harder; the quieter, individual way is more focused, more one's own, better for exploring inner bodily sensations.

For me, increasingly it was the individual path which compelled; the resistances to the outer path became too much to grapple with. Although now I see that I was right in following the individual way, at the time I battled with myself because I read the resistance as laziness, lack of discipline, weakness. Of course to some extent that was also correct—often I gave in to inertia.

Naturally, this dilemma—when to follow the natural course of least resistance and when to push against the current—did not cease to trouble me when I stopped dancing. Knowing when the ego must make a special effort to be active, when it must step aside and let nature take her course, when to force outward, when to turn in, when to be part of a group, when to focus on oneself—that is the art of energy management which "the superior man" (the anonymous sage referred to so often in the *I Ching)* may know, but which this mortal, for one, will struggle with till the end of her time on earth.

The Value of Pain

People who do not possess their center, who are somewhat outside of it, need a great deal of suffering before they can feel themselves— they almost inflict upon themselves situations in which they have to suffer. But nobody can prevent them because it is a need. Only through pain can they feel themselves, or become aware of certain things, and if they never become aware they never progress.

. . . The positive effect of it is that you feel yourself, you acquire awareness.[11]

The path to physical awareness is paved with pain; it is the constant companion of the dancer, faithful from the beginning to the end of his or her dancing days.

In his essay on marriage, Jung says that "there is no birth of consciousness without pain."[12] The dancer's experience accords with this one hundred percent. Indeed, for the dancer, it could be said that pain is the *via regia* to physical knowledge: in the effort to build a communications system, nothing establishes the telephone line between a part of the body and the brain more quickly or effectively.

I once studied with a ballet teacher, trained in the most elegant prerevolutionary Russian tradition, who quite regularly pinched her pupils. I thought this was a sadistic trait until I myself experienced the treatment. That stab of pain informed me immediately and with great precision of a muscle I had until then never realized existed. I can still feel the pinch (on the outer left side of the back at the waist) and since then that particular muscle has been a familiar colleague with whom I have undertaken many projects. My own experience tells me without any doubt that pain and memory are interconnected. I can still, twenty years later, remember where I was standing, what exercise we were working on, and that it was a sunny day outside.

Pain wakens a hitherto dormant message path—jolts it out of sleep like an electric shock. Once felt, the sensation of the muscle is connected to consciousness and can be retrieved. Over a period of time many new links between consciousness and body parts are established and the ego is able to speak to a vastly greater proportion of the body. It can begin to direct the formerly wayward body.

But this improved communications system works both ways—it is not just a matter of the ego "directing" the body; the ego that has ears to hear can learn much from the information sent over the wires.

---

[11] Jung, *The Visions Seminars*, vol. 1, pp. 126-127

[12] "Marriage as a Psychological Relationship," *The Development of Personality*, CW 17, par. 331.

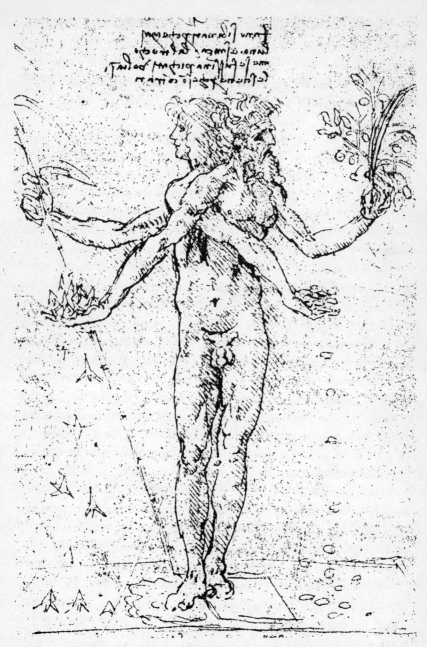

Pleasure and Pain as Twins, by Leonardo da Vinci.

Perhaps the most persistent and painful source of information about the structure of the body comes from sore, stiff muscles which have been used to excess, or in an unaccustomed way. For example, recently I tackled the weeds and brush that had grown waist-high by the side of our little dirt road. An impulse came over me to use a brush scythe.

I set out early in the morning to learn my new skill. I worked hard, albeit clumsily, for over an hour. I began to feel the rhythm, and also the satisfaction, of clearing the roadside. Finally, very weary, I returned to my desk. I immediately learned something new about energy: I was so tired physically that I could not work through the writing task I had set for the day—there was no energy left for thinking. The exhaustion of my body had drained my mind.

The following day I was extremely stiff. My shoulder muscles, particularly on the right side, were sore to the touch. My right forearm muscles hurt, but not the left. The muscles around my rib cage and waist, particularly on the left side, hurt when I moved them. My back muscles, however, did not get more use than they were prepared for, nor had my legs been heavily involved in the effort—they did not hurt.

From this and other information I knew much about what muscles I would have to develop and use if I wished to scythe more effectively for longer periods of time. In effect, my body had become a kind of map which I could read to determine how best to use my available strength and eliminate unnecessary strain.

I have described this experience at some length in order to illustrate how one can learn, from the messages sent by sore muscles, both something of the mechanisms of a physical pattern and how to refine and more efficiently execute different movements. Few dancers will be as pedantically analytical as I have been here. However, it is this sort of observation of action, reaction and redirection of effort, as a result of reading the information sent by pain, which the dancer uses to build up a working relationship with the body.

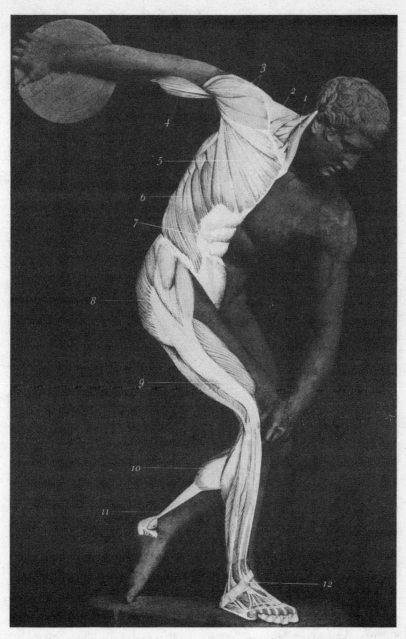

Cross-section of muscles involved in throwing the discus.

Up to this point I have been looking at pain as a fairly benign opener of communication lines, but it is of course much more complicated than that.

As I have said, muscular stiffness results from muscles being used more than they normally are; since a dancer is always trying to extend the muscles' capacities, either by trying new movements or by doing more difficult variations of familiar ones, stiffness is inevitable. But this stiffness must be managed with care. A good teacher will pace the increased use so as not to overload the student with pain, although this demands the kind of individual attention which, as I pointed out earlier, is not always possible in a class situation.

A little stiffness can be tolerated and worked out the next day—too much means the dancer can't walk or move correctly for several days and slips back severely in training. This is one reason why a student must try to work each day. A strenuous daily class causes little injury, a strenuous class once a week can be murder! Too much stiffness and pain moves into the category of injury, and instead of being helpful, stops one in one's tracks.

Heat—both physical heat and the psychological heat of constant, focused attention (working every day)—is of the greatest value in promoting growth and in minimizing the destructive aspects of physical training. The body must be warmed up gradually before it can be asked to do difficult things. Knowledgeable dancers swathe themselves in wool while practicing, even on the hottest summer day, in order to avoid sudden cooling and consequent cramping of the muscles. One works in an alchemical sweat bath to maintain a constant cooking temperature around the muscular retort.

To wash away stiffness and pain, a dancer spends a good deal of time just soaking in hot water. Heat promotes an increased circulation of blood; sweating cleanses the nerve endings blocked with lactic acid—the ashes of burnt muscle fiber. As in alchemy, it is the fiery water which washes away the impurities. For both "normal" stiffness and many injuries, one learns that heat with the consequent

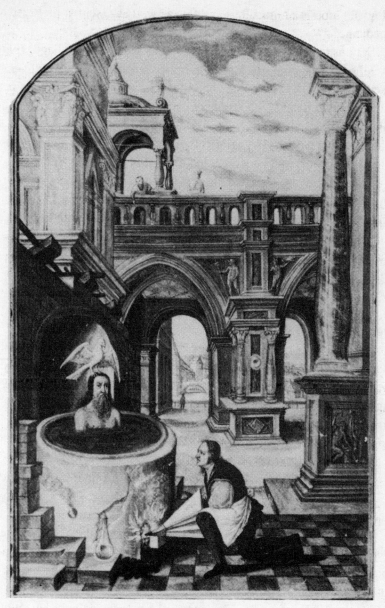

Alchemical painting of king in sweat bath.
(Trismosin, "Splendor solis," 1582)

flow of blood is a miraculous antidote as well as essential preventive medicine.

Serious injuries too—a sprained ankle, a torn knee cartilage, split Achilles tendon, ruptured spinal disc, swollen painful feet, etc.—are the frequent dark companions and teachers of a dancer. There is really nothing "natural" about the body of a dancer; its development, like psychological work on oneself, is an *opus contra naturam,* a work against nature. And nature often responds to the presumptuous efforts to improve on her creation by punishing the ego's hubris.

But you can also learn from injuries. If you sprain the right ankle, you know that the weight has been placed too far on the outside of the right foot, probably in a run or a jump. You must start again—realign the hip, the knee, strengthen the leg and foot so they can better support the force of the landing from a jump. If the crucial tendon which connects pelvis to thigh is pulled, you know you have expected too much, stretched it beyond what is physically possible; you may have to accept the fact that you cannot lift your leg as high as your fellow student.

One dancer learned an enormous amount about the structure and dynamics of the spine, especially the lower lumbar region and the sciatic nerve, because her back gave out. This was caused in part by her own individual conformation (a pronounced curvature in the lower back), an insufficient use of the abdominal muscles to hold the torso, plus an incorrect positioning of the pelvis. Above all, she had pushed too hard; the ego was greedy.

An eminent physician advised her to stop dancing altogether, and prescribed some exercises which she later discovered were exactly the wrong ones for her—they only made matters worse.

This woman couldn't entertain the idea of not dancing, so she proceeded to learn for herself the mechanics of the spine and its supporting musculature, how to use it correctly, how to heal the inflamed sciatic nerve and how to prevent a recurrence of the injury. This information considerably increased her knowledge of her own back's capabilities and limitations, and as a teacher that knowledge in turn proved of healing service to others.

All this has to do with the ethereal wonder of a Pavlova or Nijin-sky or Martha Graham—on a sensation level. Yet, it is at this con-crete anatomical level that the "heavenly" art of dance is grounded; here the vessel is built to contain the divine energy, here the archety-pal image is made flesh.

One starts out shooting for the stars—the sky's the limit, I too can be like Fonteyn! Gradually one learns, by butting up against the im-movable walls of one's physical reality, what one's limitations are. These limitations slowly coalesce into one's individual style, one's uniqueness as an expressive instrument. And often, too, one man-ages to stretch beyond what one dreamed was possible.

It works both ways, this *opus contra naturam;* like all important truths, it is a paradox. The ego's realm, "control" over the body, can be enormously enlarged, and at the same time it becomes finite. The body's possibilities are indeed limited, and soon enough the dancer learns that she cannot dictate beyond a certain point to her physical nature.

Dance training greatly expands consciousness and consequently strengthens the ego, but not in order to lord it over the body. Working in partnership with nature, as a rider does with a horse, proves to be the appropriate relationship. If one pushes beyond cer-tain boundaries or tries to go too fast, one injures one's mount and further activity is prohibited. Hence one must learn to listen, to be re-ceptive, to know how much to exert the will of the ego and when to relinquish that will to a more compelling reality.

In this connection the dancer learns to differentiate pain signals. To the careful listener, pain speaks in different timbres. A stiff mus-cle can be pushed; a short tendon stretched, but not too much. Cer-tain other sensations which also read as pain must be obeyed as a red flag to stop.

The knee, for instance, is the "unforgiving joint"—it never forgets or forgives an injury and must never be handled roughly. Some in-juries heal through working with them, others must be rested reli-giously, babied, pampered. One learns when to rest, when to push, when to wrap an ankle in a poultice of onion, when to apply ice,

when to soak in hot water, when to see a physician, and when to ignore medical advice.

One learns also that there are certain sensations that read as pain if
one approaches the area in question with a domineering, willful attitude or with fear, but which will change to a healthy stretching sensation in response to a more relaxed and friendly approach on the part
of the ego. It is as if the body, like the unconscious, reflects back the
attitude consciousness has toward it.

I used to talk to a muscle I wanted to stretch as to a frightened animal, soothing it, relaxing it, working gradually. Often I would be
rewarded by a cooperation on the part of the muscle that surprised
me. This of course is the principle behind natural childbirth which,
turning the scream of pain born of fear into more positive hard labor,
cooperates with the natural process rather than resisting it. How
often I have had a similar experience with my dog—forcing her to do
something against her will brings growls and stubbornness, whereas
a caring approach that respects her fear, her instinctive wisdom, is
more productive.

Yes, resistances, whether they be those of tight muscles, dogs or
complexes within the psyche, are to be respected.

For dancers and nondancers alike, there is meaning to be found in
the body's distress. Pain, injury, illness are voices of a starved
raven, a salmon out of water—the *lumen naturae,* nature's light.[13]
An arrogant attitude which dismisses such an encounter as "nothing
but" causes one to lose touch with the path; the fox or the bear or the
duck in fairy tales will help only the one who can slow down and
listen with lowered eyes and bowed head.

Through this kind of attention, one learns awe—awe for the
body's capacity to move, to heal, to grow, to learn, to teach, to be
stubborn, to protect itself. When this happens there is no longer an
archaic identity between ego and body; the body, the animal, becomes *other.*

---

13 See Jung, "Paracelsus as a Spiritual Phenomenon," *Alchemical Studies,*
CW 13, par. 148.

If all goes well, as one becomes two, it is partnership rather than ego willfulness which connect ego and body. In turn, ego and will are no longer identical. The ego that relates to the body in a receptive way is willing to step aside, changing from dictator to facilitator. Not the ego's desires but the design of a larger totality, the Self, of which the body is an important indicator, begins to determine the course of events. This is true, ideally, for a maturing dancer and it is certainly a mark of individuation.

Possibly, also, when the flesh is consciously connected to the ego by receptivity and relatedness, by Eros, a reunion of sorts may take place between the four sisters: Eve, Helen, Mary and Sophia.

> This thing for which you have sought so long is not to be acquired or accomplished by force or passion. It is to be won only by patience and humility, and by a determined and most perfect love.[14]

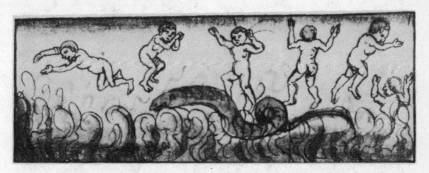

Personified *spiritus* escaping from the heated *prima materia*.
(Thomas Aquinas, "De alchimia," 16th cent.)

---

[14] Morienus, "De transmutatione metallorum," quoted in Jung, *Psychology and Alchemy,* CW 12, par. 386.

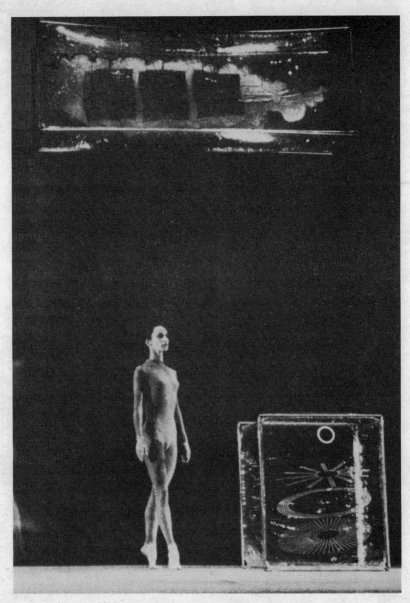

Carolyn Brown in Merce Cunningham's *Walkaround Time.*
(Photo by James Klosty)

4
Approaching the Center

[The] fundamental postulate [in the *I Ching*] is the "great primal beginning" of all that exists, *t'ai chi*—in its original meaning, "the ridge pole." . . . the line. With this line, which in itself represents oneness, duality comes into the world, for the line at the same time posits an above and a below, a right and left, front and back—in a word, the world of opposites.
—Richard Wilhelm, *The I Ching or Book of Changes.*

The Complexio Oppositorum

The way in which to organize this book came to me in a dream, in the form of a dance, .

A woman, starting at the outside corner of the stage, with a quiet stately walk and simple dance gestures circumscribed a large square, gradually spiraling into the center. There she stood and faced the audience, lifted her arms to the sky and raised her face to the sun. To me her movements represented a journey through the opposites to the center, with the dancer herself as bridge between earth and heaven.

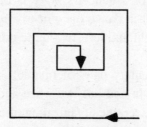

In one way or another, then, our journey thus far has been an exploration of some of the opposites in a dancer's experience.

We have touched on the polarity of the sacred, otherworldly time and space, as contrasted with "normal" time and space. We have looked at the duality of the ideal and the mundane matter of the dancer's instrument—the body as shadow. I have sketched how the original identity of body and ego gradually, through the training process, becomes two separate entities and how it seems that nature, often through pain, teaches that the ego's will and the will of the Self are not always the same.

We have explored the process of activating the inner sensation function, which plays in tandem with awareness resulting from external viewing—in the mirror, by the teacher and by the audience.

As the body wakes to consciousness the dancer learns, often through conflict, that the newly discovered internal awareness may be at odds with external demands. There is a great difference between working in the extraverted class situation and alone, at one's own tempo, focused on one's inner space.

The infinite complexity of the totality made up of opposites is clearly illustrated, to be felt and seen, in the organization and functioning of the human body. Indeed, it is a primary experience of each individual.

Running up and down both the front and back of the body, for instance, is a clearly visible central line which becomes even more obvious as the muscles gain in strength. It looks and feels just like a ridgepole, only one that runs vertically instead of horizontally. The physical organization of a dancer's body is of course no different from anyone else's, but in dance one must be *aware* of the division into front and back, right and left (two quite different personalities), and above and below.

It is with complementary pairs of functions that nature fashions each body. We breathe in and out, we wake and sleep, we stand up and lie down. For a dancer, the organization of muscles is of particular importance. To function optimally, each muscle must contract and relax alternately. The heart muscle, for instance, by rhythmic alternation of contraction and relaxation, pumps our life's blood day in and day out, as long as we live.

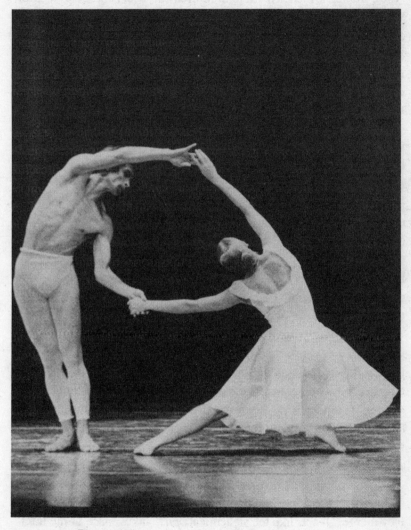

Rudolph Nureyev and Eileen Cropley in *Aureole*.
(Photo by Susan Cook)

Throughout the body, muscles are grouped in complementary pairs. To bend over, we contract the muscles of the front of the body while the back muscles stretch. To arch the back, the pattern is reversed. To lift the leg, the thigh muscles contract and the muscles at the back of the leg, the hamstrings, stretch. To lift the leg backward, the process works in reverse. Walking, running, leaping, turning, moving, grabbing something in the hand, all these and a myriad of other actions are accomplished by this constant play of opposing muscular functions.

So too, the opposites of right and left, top and bottom, are in constant alternation—spiraling—as one moves and dances. When the left leg goes forward it is naturally the right arm which goes with it; the left arm goes back. A difficult balance on one leg is held secure by, among other things, a contraction of the opposing side's shoulder blade muscle in the back. A step forward is generated by an equal amount of energy stretching behind; a jump into the air is given thrust by a strong push into the ground. Apparent stillness results from the strenuous activity of balanced energies pulling between a multitude of muscular polarities throughout the body—a pulsing tension between opposites, a living mandala.

When I was studying analytical psychology and learned that Jung felt a third world war might be avoided if enough people could stand the tension of the opposites within themselves, I was reminded of this difficult work to achieve balance within my own body. The development of the ability to continually readjust the tension connecting a hundred polarities in order to move harmoniously, as a whole, lies behind virtually all the work that goes into becoming a dancing instrument.

The following sections will explore a landscape vastly less clear, a realm where the opposites are not so easily identifiable, indeed where they merge. Dance, like the alchemical *opus,* takes place in the intermediate realm shared by matter (flesh) and spirit. Both in the training process and in the dance itself, it is at the allegorical level, the level where movement is infused with image, that we find the art, the meaning.

Image and Meaning

> Its association with the invisible forces of the psyche was the real
> secret of the *magisterium*. In order to express this secret the old mas-
> ters readily resorted to allegory.[1]

In teaching, the allegorical image is an invaluable tool. It is now generally acknowledged that the psyche can affect matter—witness psy-
chosomatic medicine—but in a day and age when psychology is all
too often reduced to a science of the brain, "nothing but" mechanics
or chemistry, it is useful to remember the extraordinary potency of
the psyche to animate the body.

An image-spark from the psychological end of the matter-psyche
spectrum, streaking to the opposite pole, can activate a sensation
which is perceived in the body, kinesthetically, as clearly as the pain
of a ballet teacher's pinch. Earlier I referred to pain as the *via regia* to
physical consciousness, but image, too, has the power to awaken a
hitherto dark corridor of communication between mind and muscle,
and image contributes not only physical awareness but quality of
movement.

For example, it is very difficult to describe to a student how to
carry the head with a fluidity and balance which is at once controlled
and free, how to find the correct position, neither too far back nor
forward, in which to balance the rather heavy mass of the skull on
the tiny uppermost bones of the spine. Physiologically the problem is
very complex and it is almost impossible to translate the solution into
words. The correct carriage is so subtle that even demonstrating how
it should look doesn't help someone whose appropriate nerve paths
are not yet awake.

Once, when I was searching for a way to get this across to a class,
the unconscious spontaneously gave me an image: "Hold your head
as if you were carrying antlers." It worked! The image, the "as if"
analogy, produced the effect I was looking for. The students could

---

[1] Jung, *Psychology and Alchemy,* par. 392.

feel the message, and I had the satisfaction of seeing fifteen beginners holding their heads correctly.

By the time a dancer begins to teach, he or she knows experien-
tially, intuitively, a great deal of physiology and anatomy, but this
knowledge is pragmatic rather than intellectual. Dancers may have
good minds but they are seldom thinking types. Their language is
predominantly physical and their verbal expression often comes in
the form of image.

Yet, an image is not simply a more archaic way of describing a
complicated chain of physical maneuvers; it is often the most concise
and efficient way, the only way. Like Kekulé's circle of dancing
atoms, an image will say it all, communicating in a flash.[2] It can induce in a student the complicated physical response no amount of
carefully detailed physiological explanation or demonstration could
convey. In fact, an image illuminates and educates a dancer much as
a dream affects the dreamer.

In teaching, helpful images often pop into one's head after one has
searched in vain for a conscious explanation. This is a mark of their
origin in the image-producing function of the psyche. They produce
an excitement in both teacher and student, a liveliness which is at
once physical and psychological. It is as if a drop of the water of life
had caused something to burst into flower, into consciousness.

The image brings color, meaning and vitality as well as physical
exactitude. It is the color and meaning which make the sensation a
memorable experience—one which ever after can be remembered and
reproduced. This, it seems to me, is thought on a preintellectual
level, where pictures rather than words represent what is not yet fully
conscious.

"Feel as if you had a third leg to balance on." "Don't let your hand
hang like a dead fish." "Move as if the space around you were heavy

---

[2] Kekulé's image-flash, which led to his discovery of the chemical structure
of the benzene ring, is often cited as an example of intuitive thinking. (See
Jung, "The Psychology of the Transference," *The Practice of Psychotherapy*,
CW 16, par. 353)

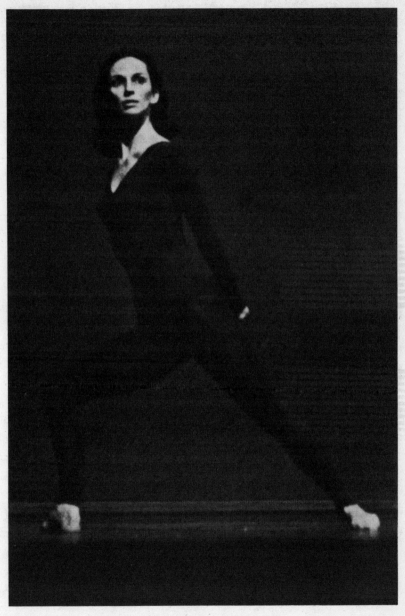

Carolyn Brown in Merce Cunningham's *Suite for Five*.
(Photo by James Klosty)

and thick. Push through it." "Listen with your cheek bones." "Your shoulder blades have eyes in them."

Each of these images conveys to the body a specific kinesthetic sensation plus a subtle, inexpressible quality. Together they develop correct movement patterns and, most importantly, evoke that special alert way of moving which belongs to a dancer. This is a quality animals have naturally, but one which human beings must work diligently to rediscover.

The Stone

> Let him study to know and to understand exactly the centre, and apply himself wholly thereto, and the centre will be freed from all imperfections and diseases, that it may be restored to its state of original monarchy.[3]

There are other images of a more profound nature. One which was of the greatest value to me, first as a student and later as a teacher, comes from Martha Graham: "Imagine you are holding a large jewel in the triangle at the base of your rib cage. Don't let it fall out!"

Physiologically this image does many things: it causes the dancer to exert just the right amount of tension in the abdominal muscles and in the muscles that hold the rib cage together. This tension prevents the ribs from caving forward or the whole torso from pulling backward in an opened "barrel" position. It encourages the dancer to stretch the upper body out of the hips, lengthening the waist, creating the proud carriage of a dancer. (After some training, a dancer may gain as much as two inches in height as a result of this "pulling up.") It also helps cast the weight of the entire body just slightly forward, and brings a physical focus into the center line of the body both vertically and horizontally.

This center point is in front of the diaphragm, the dividing muscle which controls breathing and separates the stomach from the heart

---

[3] Gerard Dorn, "De tenebris contra naturam," quoted in Jung, *Mysterium Coniunctionis,* CW 14, par. 493.

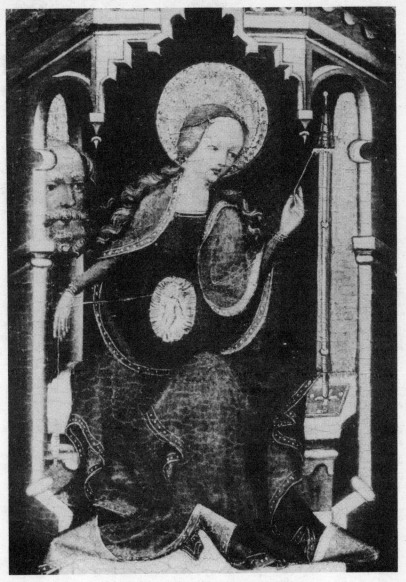

The Virgin Mary with jeweled center.
(Painting, Upper Rhenish Master, Germany, ca. 14th cent.)

and lungs. In terms of Kundalini imagery, it is midway between *manipura,* the emotional, fire chakra and *anahata,* the airy, heart chakra. It partakes of both the passion of *manipura* and the birth of objectivity which comes in *anahata.*[4]

For the Greeks, as Onians details in his study of early European thought, "thinking is described as 'speaking' and is located sometimes in the heart but usually in the *phrenes,* traditionally interpreted as 'the midriff' or 'diaphragm.' "[5] The midriff extends "roughly from just below the breast to the waistline";[6] it is effectively the center of the body. As Jung learned in his conversation with Chief Ochwiay Biano of the Taos pueblo, Indians also think from this area. From this place of the jewel comes symbolic thinking, colored and warmed by feeling.[7]

For many of us today—particularly those for whom thinking is not the primary function—it is from this mid-realm or center of the body, where thinking is not yet in the form of logical words, that image rather than word speaks. It is from here that the dancer moves. For the person used to thinking with the head, contacting this center physically lowers the thinking function back into the *phrenes,* the diaphragm, and reunites it with an earlier level of development and vitality. For the one who has yet to learn to think in a rational, differentiated way, moving or speaking from this center provides a way to communicate with others. Words come last; doing, seeing, imitating, image-making, all these come before describing.

With the beginning of objectivity, which comes through the *anahata* chakra, and the fire which burns in *manipura,* one can dance both consciously and passionately.

Graham's inspired image of holding a stone, a jewel, at this midpoint of one's being is a mark of her genius and has great psycholog-

---

[4] See Jung's psychological commentary on Kundalini yoga in *Spring 1975* (Lectures 1 & 2) and *Spring 1976* (Lectures 3 & 4).

[5] Richard B. Onians, *The Origins of European Thought,* p. 13.

[6] *American Heritage Dictionary.*

[7] See Jung, *Memories, Dreams, Reflections,* p. 248.

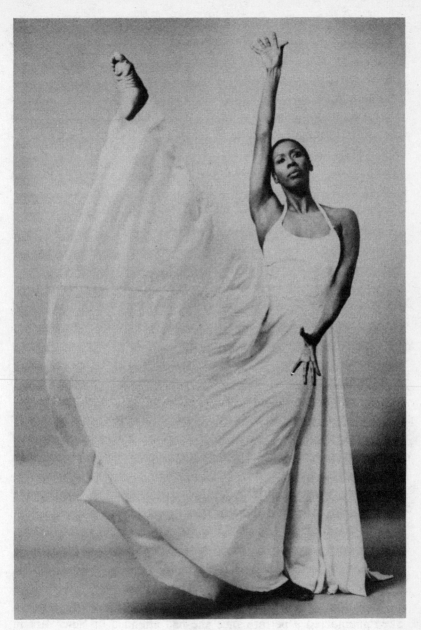

Judith Jamison.
(Photo by Jack Mitchell)

ical meaning. In the alchemical tradition, it is an image related to the philosopher's stone, the jewel of Mercury, "mediator between body and spirit."[8] Here, mind and matter, conscious and unconscious, are mysteriously joined. Clasping this center, both in one's imagination and with the various physical adjustments needed to hold the imagined stone, one moves from one's totality. Always connected to the center, the Self, one moves within a mandala. This is as true physically as it is psychologically.

In dancing, it is the ego's job to remember the image. Although the muscles, once taught, will never forget a kinesthetic sensation or how to execute a particular movement, they will, if left to their own devices, sag and droop; the stone will fall. The image will drop out of consciousness and, in both the psyche and the body, gravity's pull will prevail. In training, this image and countless others are combined to create a larger physical sensation: A+B+C+D+E+F add up to sensation, X, which becomes danced movement. The dancer learns to remember the X, the accumulation, and this becomes the physical portrait of a dancer and the message of the dance.

The Tree

If the image of the stone centers the front of the body, it is the image of the tree, the body's ridgepole, which centers the back. The back and most especially the spine, like a magnet, attracts to itself a multitude of images and provides a hook of ample proportions for psychological projections, analogies, symbols. Let us see if we can circumambulate this rich field without getting lost in its complexity.

Thus far I have illustrated the importance of images in the training process. On a larger scale, the dance is itself a picture. In the arduous process of training the body, the dancer aims to create with his or her body a moving, meaningful image.

Some time ago I was talking about the back with a friend of mine. She remembered a performance she had attended in New York in

---

8 Jung, *Mysterium Coniunctionis,* CW 14, par. 658.

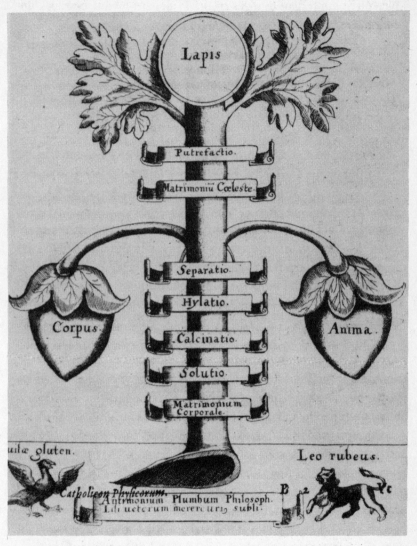

Alchemical drawing of the *arbor philosophica,* the philsophical tree,
showing stages in the transformation process.
(Samuel Norton, *Catholicon physicorum,* 1630)

which an Indian dancer performed a dance clearly inspired by the splendid South Indian bronzes of the Dancing Shiva. Heinrich Zimmer describes the dancing god thus:

> The divinity is represented as dancing on the prostrate body of a dwarfish demon. This is Apasmara Purusha, "the man or demon called. . . . Forgetfulness, or Heedlessness." It is symbolical of life's blindness, man's ignorance. Conquest of this demon lies in the attainment of true wisdom. Therein is release from the bondages of the world.[9]

I have a collection of photographs of several of these bronzes, all taken from the front. But the male dancer referred to above chose to stand with his *back* to the audience. Rooted to the spot, his feet firmly on the demon, it was with the muscles of his back that he stunningly danced the subjugation of "life's blindness, man's ignorance." My friend remembered the dance clearly and was able to pass on to me much of the power and detail of the image.[10]

Let us look at this dance for a moment from the anatomical point of view. By and large the muscles which enable the arms to move, those which initiate all lifting, reaching, holding (conscious ego work), originate in the back and are anchored to the spine. The upper back initiates and controls arm and head movement. The lower back, connected to the largest muscle mass in the body, the *maximus gluteus* or buttocks, initiates and controls movement of the legs, one's ability to move up and down, forward and backward.

With upper and lower back combined, and each divided into left and right, we have a spiraling quaternity responsible for turning the body to one side or the other or in a circle. Thus directly or indirectly, a vast proportion of movement originates in the back. Truly, as Wilhelm suggests in the passage opening this chapter, "with this line . . . duality comes into the world . . . an above and a below, a right and left, front and back— . . . the world of opposites."[11]

---

[9] *Myths and Symbols in Indian Art and Civilization,* pp. 151ff.
[10] I am indebted to Eleanor Ames Mattern for this account.
[11] Richard Wilhelm, trans., *The I Ching or Book of Changes,* p. lv.

For man and woman alike it is the front of the body with which the ego most readily identifies: "my face," "my chest," "my stomach," "my legs and feet." I look into the mirror to see what "I" look like, and it is this front which "I" present to the world, with which "I" relate to others—unless "I" wish to turn my back on them. Yet the front has a drawback: it is weak.

It was Winston Churchill's description of the Mediterranean as "the soft underbelly of Europe" that first made me aware of the vulnerability of the front of my body. Having no armor to protect it, I am one with the animals who curl up when attacked. My strength is in my back. Indeed, how odd it is that humans stand up and expose their soft, vulnerable front. Having been directed into such a singular path by nature's designers, it is no wonder that homo sapiens had to develop its wits as a shield to protect the vital organs. When I look at my dog and other four-legged animals, it seems to me their design has much to be said for it.

Now the back is quite a different proposition. First of all it is very sturdy, both in construction and function. It is less personal, less clearly identified with gender, with persona, and much less an expression of ego. In dream interpretation the back of the body can be an image of unconscious aspects of ourselves—what we don't see, what goes on "behind our backs." But this too changes for one who learns to perceive not only with the eyes, but also with the kinesthetic sense spoken of earlier.

The back is most certainly *not* insensitive, as anyone who has had a back rub will attest. What is more, a dancer begins to be able, like an animal, to sense what is going on behind his or her back. I well remember the uncanny heightened awareness I had, especially when performing, of the activity of other dancers behind me and of objects on the stage which I had to avoid bumping into. It felt as if I had eyes of a primeval variety all over my back, as if I had reconnected to the instinctual awareness that an animal has of creatures and objects unseen but not unfelt.

When trained, the back is marvelously articulated—the musculature is differentiated and sculpted, the central line of the spine strong

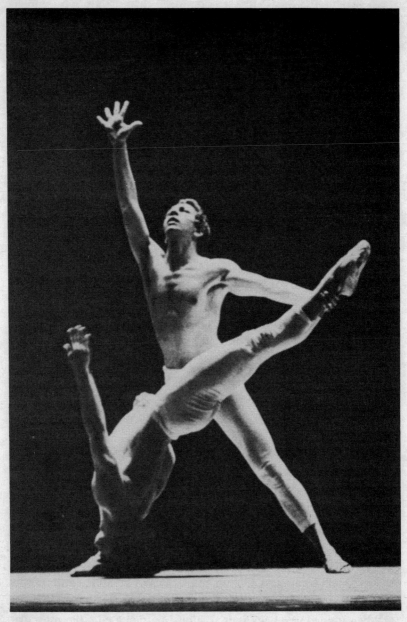

"It is the back that feels like the anchor and well-spring of movement."
(Photo by F. Peyer)

and clear. From within, a dancer senses the back as the more active plane, the front more passive. In defense of the front, it must be said that the abdominal muscles are essential to the health of the back and are capable of great effort; a chest carried correctly emits a certain light, especially when possessed of a jeweled center. Yet, in my experience, it is the back that feels, kinesthetically, like the anchor and well-spring of movement.

What psychological analogy can we draw?

One of Jung's central discoveries was that the unconscious, far from being simply a container for material repressed by the ego, is the creative matrix of consciousness, its originating source. Like the unconscious, the back, of which we are more or less unconscious in a "normal" state, is the source of most of our movement in this earthly time and space. The dancer's gradual realization of the back's strength, sensitivity and mobility, is similar on a physical plane to one's increasing awareness, as the individuation process unfolds, of the value and wonder of the unconscious as a source of life .

The physical back seems to me analogous to the layers of the unconscious closest to consciousness. Behind the physical plane lies much of a collective nature of which the ego is less aware.

I remember a most enlivening image used by one of my teachers. He told us to move as if every movement we made was only the most recent of a long chain of movements—every movement we had ever made, and our ancestors before. All this was attached to our backs and stretched out behind us.

When I heard this I felt a shock of awareness in my back. The entire surface, and the musculature beneath it, became sentient. I began to move differently. As this potent image went deeper into my being, I suddenly became aware of my place in time. The front of my body, which like the ego expresses the present and faces the future, carries on its back my personal and collective history. Even now, focusing on this image, my spine tingles.

Physiologically, the central structure of the back, the vertical ridgepole itself, is the spinal column. First let us look at it anatomically on a very simplified level.

The spine, which in man changed its earlier horizontal position to an upright one, is the key to man's ability to stand. Made of bone, it provides the scaffold and strength for this vertical posture. Anchored at the bottom, in the pelvic basin, it runs upward, a chain of bones and cartilage cushioned by shock-absorbing gelatinous discs. The whole is woven in place by a maze of tendons and muscles. The top vertebra, "carrying the head as Atlas carried the globe, is [called] the atlas. The second [vertebra] is called the axis."[12] A structural marvel, in its hollow core the spine contains and protects the main trunk of the body's communication system—the spinal cord of nerves, the lifeline of the organism.

With this vastly oversimplified description, images flood in. When I stand, the spine feels as if it were my own tree of life. I am reminded of Yggdrasil, the Norse World Tree, center of the world and source of continual regeneration and renewal. An eagle perches on its top branches, a serpent is coiled at its base and a squirrel scurries up and down the trunk carrying messages from one to the other.[13] The spinal column also stands between earth and sky; with the eagle-like intellect at the top and the serpentine sexual energies in the pelvis, the squirrel-like nerve impulses connect the opposites.

Language uses the image of the spine's upright posture to express strength, status and courage. We refer to an individual's "standing" in the world. The person who is "spineless," with "no backbone," is a coward.

As the central axis of the skeleton, the spine provides structural strength for both psyche and body. It enables us to "stand up" to difficulties, "straight as an arrow." Anyone who has suffered a bad back knows all too well how debilitating that is. One is no longer upright, or able to walk. "To bed with you," says the doctor, and the patient is indeed "flat on his back," immobilized. When the spine heals, the patient is "back on his feet."

---

[12] Fritz Kahn, *The Human Body,* p. 94. I quote this because it shows how scientific nomenclature is still informed by mythological analogy.

[13] H.R. Ellis Davidson, *Gods and Myths of Northern Europe,* pp. 190-196.

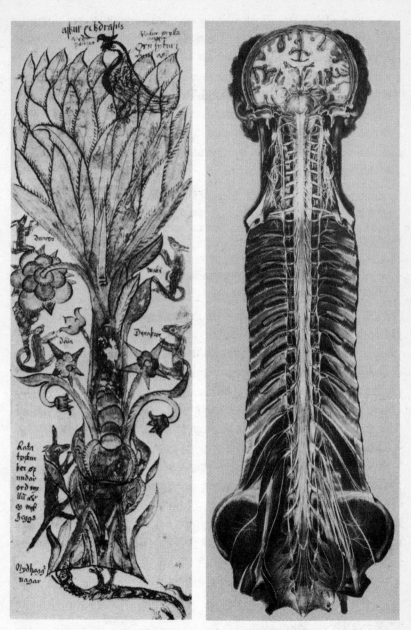

Left: Yggdrasil, Norse World Tree.
Right: the spinal column, central cable of the nervous system.

In the realm of the flesh, the spine is analogous to rod, pole or staff, all symbols of power, of ruling. The bishop's staff is a sign of his connection to the *axis mundi*—the cosmic ridgepole, so to speak—wherein resides the strength and authority of the Almighty. This too is a variation of the World Tree.

The spine's series of vertebrae joined vertically suggest ascending and descending. I am reminded again of the tree, this time the shaman's tree, his ladder, by means of which he climbs to heaven and descends to the underworld.

Initiation into the third and highest shamanic degree of the Sarawak *manang* includes a ritual climb. A great jar is set on the veranda with two small ladders leaning against its sides. Facing each other, the two initiatory masters make the candidate climb up one of the ladders and down the other throughout a whole night. . . . Its meaning seems clear enough; it must represent a symbolic ascent to the sky followed by a return to earth.[14]

The spine, connecting as it does the lowest center, the sexual generative energy, to the upper reaches of the mind, links physical life to intellectual life, concrete matter to disembodied spirit. Like the shamanic ladder or tree, it connects the depth of the earth to the high reaches of heaven. The spinal ladder transverses the middle realm of being, the trunk of the tree, the trunk of the body, a human life span. This physiological fact is the concrete base for the symbolism of Kundalini yoga.

In his seminar on the subject, Jung said that "Kundalini yoga in its systems of chakras symbolizes the development of that impersonal life, therefore it is at the same time an initiation symbolism, and it is the cosmogonic myth."[15] It symbolizes the individuation process as experienced through the body's image-suggesting facts.

Chakra imagery, related as it is to the series of nerve ganglia "arranged in two chains along the spinal column,"[16] leads us from

---

14 Mircea Eliade, *Shamanism,* p. 126.
15 *Spring 1975,* p. 23.
16 Kahn, *The Human Body,* p. 203.

the structural, skeletal aspect of the spine to its role as conductor, container and protector of the spinal cord.

From earliest times the spinal cord, also called the spinal marrow, was believed to contain the stuff of life.

> There is evidence that the life-soul was particularly associated not only with the brain but with the whole of the cerebro-spinal "marrow." Through the vertebrae "the marrow descends from the brain . . . ." Thus Pliny; and there is evidence a good deal earlier that for the Romans the marrow was the stuff of vitality and strength.[17]

The spinal marrow or spinal cord is not merely an analogy for the life process; it is, concretely, a central ingredient thereof. Both the central nervous system, which governs the motor and sensory functions, and the autonomic nervous system, which directs the digestive and circulatory systems, depend upon the communication network in and around the spinal cord.

In modern medicine, the functions of a great many organs and glands can be taken over, at least for a time, by machines or pills. A life-support system can keep a person clinically alive, but nothing can replace a severed spinal cord. It is no wonder that for the Greeks, "to divide the 'spinal marrow' at the neck [was] the most expeditious way of rendering unconscious and killing."[18]

Onians contributes yet another piece of information to the intricate maze of associations to the spine. Not only the substance of life, but also that which remains after death seems to dwell in the spinal cord:

> It was, we found, more particularly with the cerebro-spinal marrow that the psyche, the life-soul that lives on after death, was associated. This is confirmed by and throws light upon two other beliefs which we may now put together: (I) that . . . a dead man's psyche assumes snake form—it was represented thus at tombs—a belief which lingered on chiefly in association with the mighty dead, i.e. "heroes"; and (2) that the spinal marrow of a dead man turns into a snake.[19]

---

[17] Onians, *Origins of European Thought*, p. 149.
[18] Ibid., p. 206.
[19] Ibid.

With the appearance of the serpent, the psyche-snake, it is but a short step to the Kundalini serpent, and also to the frequent image of the serpent as the spirit within the tree. Perhaps the most familiar example of this in Western culture is the snake in the Biblical Garden of Eden.

Thrown out of paradise, the snake later migrated to the alchemical laboratory, where it became associated with all manner of life-giving processes. Most prominently, it is a symbol of the vital energy of the psyche which, contained in physical matter and intimately connected to the nervous system, flows up and down the body, animating and transforming the human being.[20]

The dancer who chose to illustrate with his back the process of growth which comes out of the effort to trample underfoot Apasmara Purusha, used the most powerful plane of his body. By presenting his back to the audience he was able to demonstrate the tremendous strength, activity, steadfastness and timelessness inherent not in the ego but in the less personal aspect of the psyche that becomes activated in the effort to subdue the demon of ignorance. This effort we call the individuation process. It is the vitality and power of the Self, not the ego, which this dance represents to me—the vitality and courage of a lifetime and beyond, passing through us from our ancestral past and forward into an unknown future.

Shiva's dance on the animal demon is an image of the effort to move consciousness above the animal level of blind existence. Similarly, in the Christian world there has historically been a concerted effort to tame the animal instincts, an effort symbolized in medieval sculpture by images of Christ standing on beasts or demons—subjugating the raw forces of nature.[21] The attempt to spiritualize human nature is strongly associated in the Western psyche with that

---

[20] As a symbol of the individuation process in a human lifetime, the serpent leads to that mysterious possibility, the subtle body, which may remain after death when the physical body sinks back into the earth. See Jung, *Nietzsche's Zarathustra*, esp. pp. 441ff.

[21] See James Snyder, *Medieval Art*, especially pp. 190 (the Ruthwell Cross), 369-370 (Chartres Cathedral) and 378 (Amiens Cathedral).

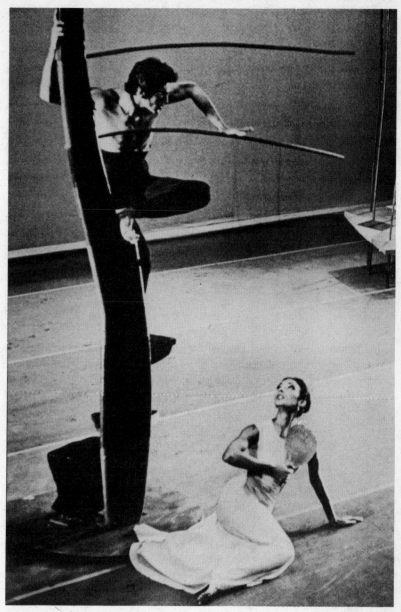

Robert Cohan as the stranger (serpent) and Matt Turney as Lilith
in Martha Graham's *Embattled Garden*.
(Set by Isamu Noguchi; photo by Martha Swope)

central symbol of Christianity, the crucifixion, which in turn is related, though not in an immediately obvious way, to spinal imagery.

This connection was made in a dream brought to me by a dancer in her mid-forties. In the dream she was standing on the ground in a meadow to the left of the cross on which Christ was nailed. The cross and Christ appeared in profile. It was clear to the dreamer that Christ's backbone and the vertical member of the cross (a stout square beam of wood) were contiguous—in psychological language, analogous. It was, she felt, as if the man's spine drew its strength from the thick piece of wood, his tree of life.

It is worth noting that the spine is not buried within the flesh of the body but is on the surface of the back. Representing a link between the ego and the objective psyche, the spine connects to and draws strength from the archetypal characteristics of the tree:

> Taken on average, the commonest associations to [the tree's] meaning are growth, life, unfolding of form in a physical and spiritual sense, development, growth from below upwards and from above downwards, the maternal aspect (protection, shade, shelter, nourishing fruits, source of life, solidity, permanence, firm-rootedness, but also being "rooted to the spot"), old age, personality, and finally death and rebirth.[22]

An individual who has backbone, who is connected to the ancestral cosmic tree and carries on his or her back, for a time, the task of life, must suffer the pain of holding together the opposites—a veritable crucifixion.

The vertical direction, emphasized in the above dream, implies an energetic tension between instinct and mind, the growth through time from the purely instinctual to the conscious living of life. But the process must be rooted. While Shiva dances close to earth, in the crucifixion Christ is lifted off the ground. This elevation represents the two thousand year long effort at spiritualization.[23]

---

[22] "The Philosophical Tree," *Alchemical Studies*, CW 13, par. 350.
[23] See Jung, *Psychology and Religion*, CW 11, pars. 310, 317.

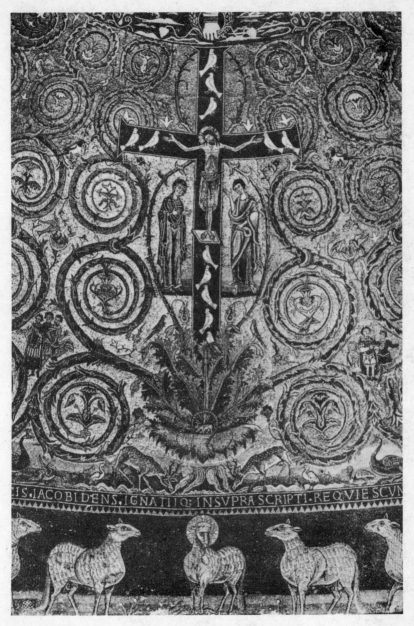

The cross as Tree of Life.
(Church of S. Clemente, Rome, 12th cent.)

This elevated ideal—more fully realized of late in the development of our intellectual factulties than in our spiritual life—has tended to cut us off from a conscious connection to physical nature. As with Christ, our relationship to the maternal aspect of nature has perforce been kept behind our back, in the unconscious. That this arrangement is changing is expressed in many ways, among which, as mentioned earlier, is the increased interest in physical activities.

Just as Mary must be allowed to come down to earth, so too must Christ be brought closer to the ground, separate from, though still related to, the tree behind him.

Paralleling Jung's experience on the Athi Plains,[24] the woman in the dream above, feet planted on the ground, by her witnessing brings the tree-man god down to her mortal standpoint. By observing the difficult archetypal drama taking place she also takes part in it— realizes it, incarnates it. This means she must live the opposites within herself. In outer life she was a woman who had conscious knowledge of her body; from it she could draw strength.

In a way we are all the gods'—the archetypes'—tree of life; with our bodies, lives consciously lived, we ground the gods and provide for them a human vessel in which to be transformed. This is, I believe, one of the ways in which we can assist the *coniunctio* of masculine and feminine, spirit and matter, consciousness and the unconscious.

The cross, the ladder, the transformation process, are one and the same. Each is sturdy only when firmly planted in the ground, in a human life. "You see the shoot must come out of the ground, and if the personal spark has never gotten into the ground, nothing will come out of it."[25] But it must be consciously planted; until then we are possessed by matter and mother *(mater)*, not related to it. Relationship is impossible when there is unconscious identity.

The case of a clergyman illustrates the problem. When he entered analysis he was having severe back trouble; the upper part of his

---

[24] See *Memories, Dreams, Reflections,* pp. 255-256.
[25] Jung, "Kundalini Yoga," *Spring 1975,* p. 22.

spine was painfully rigid and continually out of alignment at the shoulders and neck. This gave him a constant headache. Before his first hour he dreamed that he was caught up in a tree, unable or at least afraid to come down. Underneath the tree was a bull who had two front feet up on the tree's trunk. The bull was not angry, and indeed seemed friendly, as if, the dreamer thought, he wanted the dreamer to come down and become acquainted.

This man, like many others with a strong mother complex, was hung up in the maternal aspect of the tree and in the maternal institution of the church. He was, in Jung's words, "still connected by an umbilical cord as thick as a ship's rope with the pleroma, the archetypal world of splendour."[26] His masculine energy (the bull) invited him to come down to earth and make friends, but he dared not accept the responsibility for living out that power. His body and his head were separated, and so his body became a painful and autonomous complex.

At first he relied on a chiropractor to do his physical work for him. As time went on, however, he began to work out himself in the gymnasium, strengthening and getting to know his body, his bull. He came to accept it and in fact to enjoy its power, and as he did so his spinal disorder cleared up. The mother-bound energy, instead of crippling his neck, moved down into his body. He began to dare to live his earthly shadow, with courage and determination, and gradually ceased to be a prisoner of the maternal tree—his misaligned spine.

Today, many years after I stopped dancing, the only physical exercises I still do with any degree of regularity are those to keep my spine strong and flexible. A healthy spine is not "ramrod stiff." (Psychologically, that would point to a rigid attitude.) It must be able to curve forward and arch back, to turn at each vertebra from side to side, to move like a serpent, and each vertebra must be correctly related to the one above and below it.

---

[26] Ibid., p. 21.

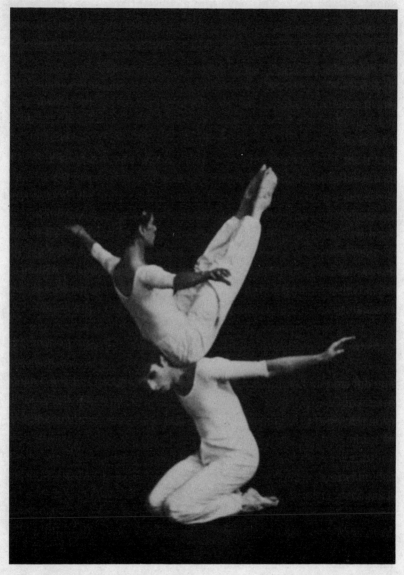

Ruxandra Racovitza and Gheorge Caciuleanu in *Founambulis*.
(Photo by Pierre Petitjean)

My ritual of stretches and contractions has both physiological and psychological value. Kinesthetically I know when my spine is out of alignment; it feels uncomfortable and deadened, the physical energy doesn't flow properly. Psychologically, like all ritual, the effect of the exercises is to gather my psychic energy and turn it inward, making contact with the wisdom of the unconscious at my back, the *lumen naturae,* without which I am unable to work.

The physical reality feels good, the psychological reality and imagery makes creative work possible. The sap of the tree, the water of life, begins to flow, or at least to trickle. I am connected to the *axis mundi*—"thy rod and thy staff, they comfort me."[27]

In the front of our bodies we are centered by the stone; at the back, by the tree. The tree and the *lapis,* both central images of alchemy, are still alive and vibrating, center and source of movement, creating the cross of our bodies on which we hang our souls for the journey through life.

> "Thus the stone is perfected of and in itself. For it is the tree whose branches, leaves, flowers, and fruits come from it and through it and for it, and it is itself whole or the whole . . . and nothing else." Hence the tree is identical with the stone and, like it, a symbol of wholeness.[28]

---

[27] Psalms 23:4, King James version.
[28] Jung, "The Philosophical Tree," *Alchemical Studies,* CW 13, par. 423 (quoting from *Ars chemica*).

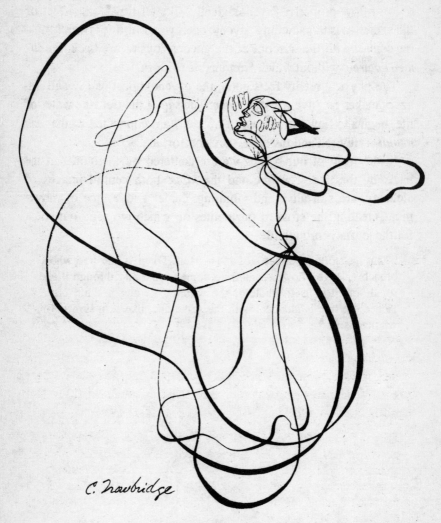

C. Trowbridge

Martha Graham.

5
Transformation of Energy

Symbols act as *transformers*, their function being to convert
libido from a "lower" into a "higher" form.
—C.G. Jung, *Symbols of Transformation.*

The transformation of libido through the symbol is a process
that has been going on ever since the beginnings of humanity
and continues still. Symbols were never devised consciously,
but were always produced out of the unconscious by way of
revelation or intuition.
—C.G. Jung, "On Psychic Energy."

Rhythm and Geometry

In speaking of the chest and the spinal column as stone and tree,
symbols of wholeness, we have moved into the symbolic realm, the
realm where natural instinctual energy can evolve from concrete to
less concrete expression.

Jung illustrates the transformative value of symbol in his description of the spring fertility dance ceremony performed by the
Wachandi of Australia:

They dig a hole in the ground, oval in shape and set about with
bushes so that it looks like a woman's genitals. Then they dance
around this hole, holding their spears in front of them in imitation
of an erect penis. As they dance round, they thrust their spears into
the hole, shouting: "Pulli nira, pulli nira, wataka!" (not a pit, not a
pit, but a c—!). During the ceremony none of the participants is allowed to look at a woman.

By means of the hole the Wachandi make an analogue of the female genitals, the object of natural instinct. By the reiterated shouting and the ecstasy of the dance they suggest to themselves that the

95

hole is really a vulva, and in order not to have this illusion disturbed by the real object of instinct, none may look at a woman. There can be no doubt that this is a canalization of energy and its transference to an analogue of the original object by means of the dance . . . and by imitating the sexual act.

. . . The Wachandi's hole in the earth is not a sign for the genitals of a woman, but a symbol that stands for the idea of the earth woman who is to be made fruitful. . . . It is for this reason that none of the dancers may look at a [real] woman.[1]

With dance, then, instinct in its raw form (often sexual in character) can be channeled to productive and cultural goals—that is, spiritualized. In this process, as Marie-Louise von Franz points out, rhythm plays an extremely important role:

All emotional, and therefore energy-laden, psychic processes evince a striking tendency to become rhythmical. . . . This fact presumably also explains the basis of various rhythmical and ritual activities practiced by primitives. Through them, psychic energy and the ideas and activities bound up with it are imprinted and firmly organized in consciousness. It also explains the dependence of work-achievement on music, dancing, singing, drumming, and rhythm in general; through such means a restraint on uncoordinated instinctuality is achieved. The application of rhythm to psychic energy was probably the first step toward its cultural formation, and hence toward its spiritualization.[2]

All dance is timed and rhythmical. Sometimes the rhythm is intuitive, free-flowing, built on phrases of breath, of rise and fall, of increase and decrease in intensity.

Even more frequently, in dance highly crafted as an art form, rhythm is metrically organized, carefully counted. Counting not only organizes dance in time but takes the movement out into space: every gesture, every pause, every step in any direction is placed in a rhythmical, numbered phrase.

---

[1] "On Psychic Energy," *The Structure and Dynamics of the Psyche,* CW 8, pars. 83-84, 88.
[2] *Number and Time,* pp. 157-158.

In *Number and Time,* von Franz explores the qualitative aspect of number.[3] The permeation of dance with number provides a useful illustration of these qualities. To the dancer, it is evident that each of the simple numbers—one, two, three, four, five—has its own special character. *One* begins, grounds, holds. The strength given to the accented *one,* the first of a group of beats, suggests the sum total of energy, the intensity of the movement.

The polarity of *two* is obvious in the alternation of right and left feet, in walking, running and other locomotion. The basic balanced experience of *right*-left, *right*-left (*RL, RL, RL, RL*) is quite different from the dynamic, driving intensity of *three,* a triplet (*RLR, LRL, RLR, LRL*). *Three* never quite comes to rest; the dancer always wants to take yet one more step to balance the previous one, always seeking and never reaching the completion of four.

In teaching, when a class becomes slow and needs more energy, putting the exercise on a rhythm of three immediately accelerates the energy level. In playing music or singing, one easily experiences the rushing—it is difficult to keep a triplet rhythm (especially a 6/8 meter) from speeding up, while a two or a four rhythm keeps its tempo more steadily.

The wholeness, completeness, of *four* permeates all rhythmic organization. A grouping of four beats is the most common and instinctual form of phrasing, of rhythmic sentence making. Most dance exercises form themselves into phrases of four or eight groups of four, often ending with a hold on the quintessential *five* or *nine.*[4]

It is difficult to put this qualitative aspect of rhythm into words but give me a drum and some open space and I could show you in a trice. The first-hand experience of danced number, felt deeply in the body, has been for me an extremely rich source of amplification of numbers in dreams and other unconscious material.

---

[3] Ibid., esp. chapters 4-7.

[4] Cf. the "axiom of Maria Prophetissa," a central tenet of alchemy: "One becomes two, two becomes three, and out of the third comes the one as the fourth." (Jung, *Psychology and Alchemy,* par. 26)

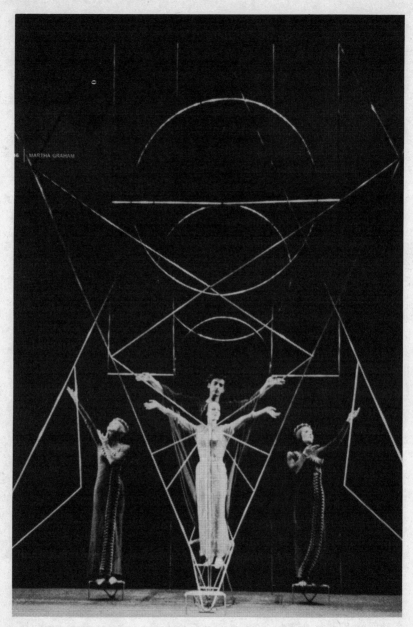

The Martha Graham Company in Graham's *Seraphic Dialogue.*
(Set by Isamu Noguchi; photo by Martha Swope)

In space, dance is organized by using countless combinations of basic geometric elements. Straight lines, angles, diagonals, triangles, squares, crosses, circles, spirals . . . these familiar patterns of the psyche provide the spatial structure for the danced image. Anyone who has had the fun of folk-dancing has, with his or her feet, traced an infinite variety of mandalas. Simple and instinctive, these peasant dances mirror the dance of the psyche, of the cosmos. The choreographer uses the same handful of elementary geometric elements to construct an evening-long ballet.

At a dance performance, I like to sit in the balcony. From there one can see the marvelous elaboration of geometric patterns, the moving canvas the dancers paint on the stage. This image is visible for but a fleeting moment, and, like life's pattern, remains afterward only in the memory, ringing a responsive vibration in the psyche.

In both natural and highly conscious dance, the fundamental organizing element which lies beneath rhythm and spatial design is number, "the very element which regulates the unitary realm of psyche and matter."[5] As von Franz notes:

[Number] throws a bridge across the gap between the physically knowable and the imaginary. In this manner it operates as a still largely unexplored midpoint between myth (the psychic) and reality (the physical), at the same time both quantitative and qualitative, representational *and* irrepresentational. . . . It preconsciously orders both psychic thought processes *and* the manifestations of material reality.[6]

If the symbol acts as transformer, we might say that number, in one form as rhythm, another as geometrical shape, provides the stones which pave the channel to direct and order the flow of energy from lower to higher, concrete to symbolic.

Providing, as I believe it might, an accessible example of the "unitary reality underlying the dualism of psyche and matter,"[7] the

[5] Ibid., p. 27.
[6] Ibid., p. 52.
[7] Ibid., p. 171.

place of danced number invites further study. Perhaps dance could provide an experience with which to amplify, for those not trained in mathematics, some of the complex ideas von Franz has explored in this field.

Suffice it for now to say (though it is hardly sufficient) that every movement a dancer makes, in training and in performance, is made manifest, temporally and spatially, through the organizing power of number. Image brings symbolic meaning into dance, but it is number which orders it and places it in three-dimensional reality.

The "Extraordinarily Potent"[8]

> My personal view in this matter is that man's vital energy or libido is the divine pneuma.[9]

Dance is a direct expression of how libido, "vital energy," may manifest in human life. The energy itself is neutral, "able to communicate itself to any field of activity whatsoever, be it power, hunger, hatred, sexuality, or religion."[10] The essential question, then, is to what end is the energy involved in dance directed? Where does the channel lead?

Dance, and particularly rhythm, can release energy or it can bind it. It can allow it to flood, or direct it to a specific goal. Rhythm itself has the power not only to channel energy toward consciousness but to possess the personality completely and send it into deep unconsciousness. Curt Sachs, the dance historian, writes:

---

8 "The creative mana, the power of healing and fertility, the 'extraordinarily potent' . . . [has] equivalents in mythology and in dreams [such as] the bull, the ass, the pomegranate, the yoni, the he-goat, the lightning, the horse's hoof, the dance, the magical cohabitation in the furrow, and the menstrual fluid, to mention only a few . . . . That which underlies all the analogies . . . is an archetypal image whose character is hard to define, but whose nearest psychological equivalent is perhaps the primitive mana-symbol." (Jung, "The Practical Use of Dream-Analysis," *The Practice of Psychotherapy,* CW 16, par. 340)

9 Jung, *Letters,* p. 384 (to Father Victor White, Oct. 1945).

10 Jung, *Symbols of Transformation,* par. 197.

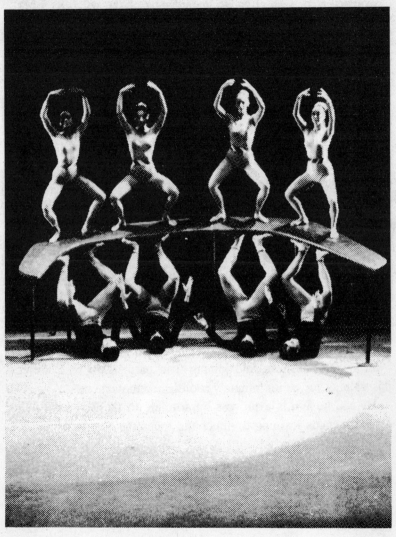
Martha Graham's *Acrobats of God.*
(Set by Isamu Noguchi; photo by Martha Swope)

The most essential method of achieving the ecstatic is the rhythmic beat of every dance movement. As anyone can testify from his own experience, it is an effective unburdening of the will. [As Beck writes] "The movements are executed automatically without the intervention of the self. Thus the consciousness of self disappears completely and is lost in the primitive consciousness. Rhythmic motion has become therefore the carrier of almost every ecstatic mood of any significance in human life."[11]

It is not surprising that the shaman's drum is called his horse, nor that in Siberia the shaman's trance is often induced by dancing.[12]

In *The Owl Was a Baker's Daughter,* Marion Woodman gives a good example of dance used as a releasing experience, one which can melt the overrational ego and reconnect it to the freeing and healing energy of the unconscious.[13] For many, this can be a very important experience. Here, however, I am focusing on the opposite process—the use of dance as a tool with which to direct libido to consciousness.

The training I have described results in a highly disciplined, narrowly focused, goal-oriented dancer. This kind of work fashions a technically exact instrument which is not for "free expression," nor for "interpretive dance." Its goal is certainly not to release repressed emotions. Separating, as it does, the body with its instinctual energy from unconsciousness, and joining it in partnership with the ego, this training strives for minutely coordinated movement.

By and large it is a process appropriate to the first half of life, when the ego is learning to direct and focus the energy which is, or could be, at its disposal.

Dancing requires a tremendous amount of physical energy. It is a path chosen by those who have a particularly strong current rushing through them, a Dionysian flow which threatens to overwhelm—"the extraordinarily potent" in full force. Those who wish to use this en-

---

[11] Curt Sachs, *World History of the Dance,* p. 25 [quoting Beck, *Die Ekstase* (Sachsa, 1906), p. 10.]

[12] Mircea Eliade, *Shamanism,* pp. 174ff.

[13] *The Owl Was a Baker's Daughter,* pp. 111ff.

ergy, rather than be swept away by it, must build an especially strong container within themselves to hold and employ what Walter F. Otto, in his study of Dionysus, calls "the maddening desire to dance."[14]

The following excerpts from interviews with three well-known and successful dancers will illustrate what I mean.

> My mother first took me to ballet classes when I was four because I had a lot of energy. I think she had a really hard time keeping it channeled in the right direction so that I didn't run over the furniture and break things.[15]

> My mother complained that I was almost hyperactive—I wouldn't eat, wouldn't sleep and was always restless. The doctor said, "Well, we will have to tire her out . . . why don't you have her study some sort of dancing?"[16]

> I'm not taking class next week. . . I know the body needs rest, so I will force myself to take that rest, and then by the end of the week I'll be taking class again. . . . I get shaky like a junkie. And I have to get that energy out. Only work does it for me. . . . I tried to take a three-month vacation in Jamaica last year, but I turned around and flew back after three days. I was going crazy. I couldn't keep still. I still have that kind of energy I had when I was a kid. I guess I was what they'd call hyperactive now.[17]

The discipline of dance is admirably suited to direct such a charge of energy. The physical discipline demands and uses great energy and endurance; the symbolic content of the dance moves it to a higher level. After the time of training is completed, the body can be used vigorously as an instrument through which the gods can sing of the archetypal patterns of existence.

There comes a time for all dancers, however, when the enormous amount of energy needed to embody the archetypal images is more

---

14 *Dionysus: Myth and Cult,* p. 81.

15 Martine van Hamel, prima ballerina, American Ballet Theater, quoted in Cynthia Lyle, *Dancers on Dancing,* p. 12.

16 Violette Verdy, prima ballerina, New York City Ballet, ibid., p. 62.

17 Judith Jamison, lead dancer, Alvin Ailey Co., ibid., p. 97.

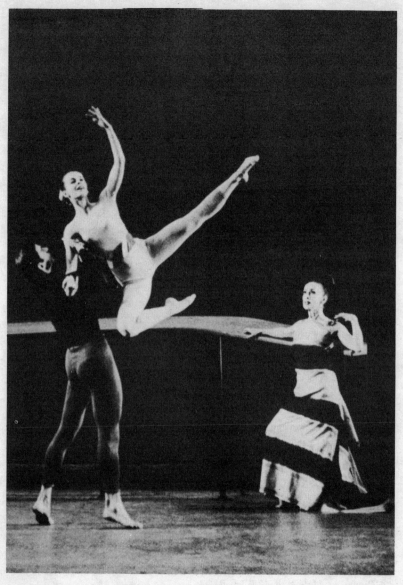

"Those who are gifted choreographers can pass on their movements
to other, younger bodies."
(Martha Graham with Bert Ross and Ethel Winters
in *Acrobats of God;* photo by Martha Swope)

than the physical vessel, with its natural aging process, can sustain. When this time comes, if the individual psyche is to continue its ascent while the body declines, the process of expressing the divine energy must continue to manifest itself symbolically in a less concrete, more energy-efficient mode.

This is a painful and sad transition for a dancer. One must sacrifice one's role as an athlete of the gods. It requires nothing less than the acceptance of mortality—acknowledging the reality of the body's death. I doubt very much if many dancers make this sacrifice consciously; I do know of one dancer who consciously chose death rather than a life without dancing. Those who are gifted choreographers can pass on their movements to other, younger bodies. Others must learn, if they can, to dance in other ways.

In alchemy much time and effort is given to the purification of the *prima materia*. In the alchemical *opus* of dance training, the same work goes into cleansing the human body of unconsciousness. For the alchemist this was performed on inanimate matter; the dancer works on his or her own body. There is no split between the dance adept and the material on which he or she performs the operations of dissolving, cleansing, heating and reshaping. "The body with its darkness . . . [is] 'prepared.' "[18] When the matter of the body is made conscious, the divine pneuma can be released from its containment in flesh.

No longer identified with the body, no longer totally dependent upon the body as its vehicle, the spirit is free, if such is the individual's fate, to dance onward psychologically.

In the training of a woman dancer, it is the animus that is the active aspect; it provides the focusing, the discipline, the goal-directed nature of the *opus*. I am reminded of the two acrobats in the dream with which we began this circumambulation. Through the training process and with the activity of the acrobats, Mercurius as the principle of individuation is crystallized, ready to serve as psychopomp, to turn the wheels of transformation for the second stage of the *opus*—

---

18 Jung, *Mysterium Coniunctionis,* CW 14, par. 774.

the inner journey. This suggests that dance training can promote the development and subsequent release of a differentiated, spiritual animus.

For a man, ideally the result of the training process would be the transformation of the anima, his inner woman. It would parallel more closely the work of the male alchemists—redemption of the feminine soul from matter. The process for a man is complicated, however; the fact that the male dancer is a consort of the Great Mother may make the separation from her especially difficult.

For men and women alike, a central aspect of the *opus* is that matter itself is redeemed, brought into the light from behind the curtain of darkness which Christianity erected. Eve and Helen are released from instinctive physicality. The acrobat-dancer builds the staircase down which the spiritual aspects of the *Sapientia Dei*—Mary and Sophia—can descend within the individual. Thus brought down to earth, into reality, they can join with their bodily sisters. No longer moved by the instinctual form of the divine pneuma, the body can with more consciousness live more wisely, a vessel in which feminine wisdom can walk upon the earth.

In this way does dance help to heal the split in the feminine which Christianity, albeit by necessity, brought about.

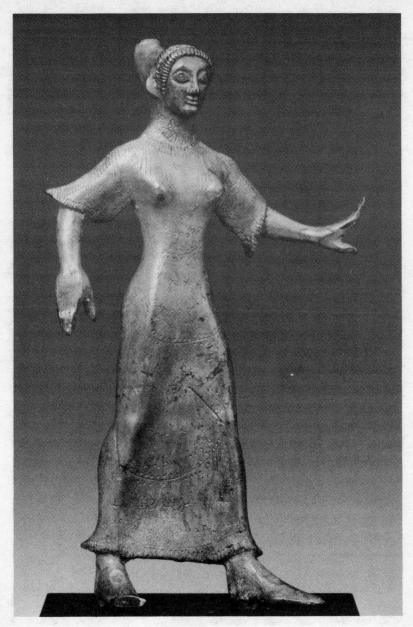

Woman dancing.
(Bronze, Etruscan, ca. 500 B.C.; Museum of Fine Arts, Boston)

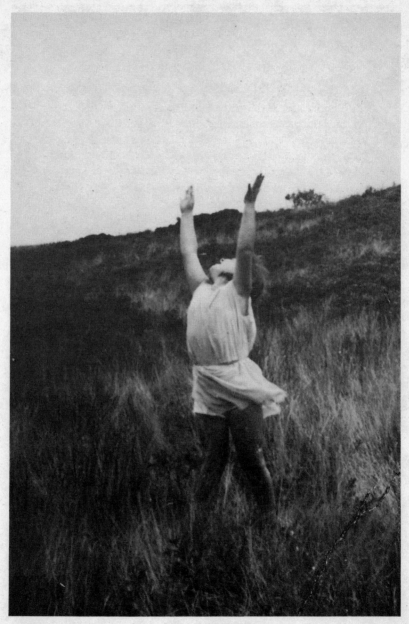

"To receive the energy of earth, of nature, and send it up to heaven . . . letting it course through the body . . . that is the ministry of a dancer."

Conclusion

If we can reconcile ourselves to the mysterious truth that the spirit is the life of the body seen from within, and the body the outward manifestation of the life of the spirit—the two being really one—then we can understand why the striving to transcend the present level of consciousness through acceptance of the unconscious must give the body its due, and why recognition of the body cannot tolerate a philosophy that denies it in the name of the spirit.

—C.G. Jung, "The Spiritual Problem of Modern Man."

Martha Graham once likened the life of a dancer to that of a nun. Man or woman, one must be called, and he or she who answers the call lives a cloistered life. There is little room in a professional dancer's life for anything but the work.

Announcing his retirement from the stage, the great dancer Eric Bruhn summed up his feelings about his twenty-six-year career as follows:

It's been a long love affair—so passionate that it has taken all my time. Being old-fashioned, I haven't had time for another affair. It was a love-hate affair that goes on and on. Now it has stopped. I feel relieved. I have a freedom I have not known or wanted until now.[1]

It seems to me that professional dancers, like the medieval juggler Barnabas, are members of a vestigial religious order. It is the Great Mother in her many forms whom they serve: they are hers and through them her natural wisdom, her energy, flows. In them it is transformed; by it they are transformed. To receive the energy of earth, of nature, and send it up to heaven—to stand with arms upstretched to receive the spiritual energy of the sun, letting it course

---

[1] Quoted by Anna Kisselgoff, *New York Times,* 1971.

through the body to bring its fertilizing spirit down to an awakened earth—that is the ministry of a dancer.

But what about the laity? Priests and priestesses are not the only humans to serve thus. The professionals may act as mediators, examples of service, but the lay members also worship, may also serve. As audience, yes, to witness the performance of the rites, but now many are asking to partake in the service itself, giving if not total dedication at least more than passive witness. Much can be gained and given by individuals who would learn to know and use their bodies consciously. They too can experience the joy and hardship of being the medium through which divine energy can both transform and be itself transformed.

What does this mean for depth psychology?

In his commentary on Kundalini yoga, Jung speaks eloquently of the importance of being securely born in the world of reality.

> You must believe in this world, make roots, do the best you can, even if you have to believe in the most absurd things—to believe, for instance, that this world is very definite, that it matters absolutely whether such and such a treaty is made or not. It may be completely futile, but you have to believe in it, have to make it an almost religious conviction, merely for the purpose of putting your signature under the treaty, as it were, so that that trace is left of you. For you should leave some trace in this world, something which notifies the world that you have been here. If nothing happens of this kind, you have not realized yourself.[2]

If one is not born into this world, if one remains suspended in the pleroma, if one is not at home in one's own body, one must at some point return to the beginning, to the place where body and psyche are identical, and plant one's psychic seed in the earth of the body. The fundamental joining of this world and the other world must take place. It is this process which I believe can be aided by, and is ultimately the purpose behind, a person's involvement with physical activity.

---

[2] *Spring 1975,* pp. 21-22.

In a course of therapy, then, it is sometimes appropriate to support hints from the psyche for such a grounding impulse—to encourage some physical discipline.

A young man who was not yet grounded in life worked with me for some time analytically. Together we succeeded to some extent in planting him in reality. Still, the hours with him were marked by manifestations of intense physical energy: rubbing of eyes, fast foot-tapping, pacing and so on. We spoke often of this pent-up energy but he avoided dealing with it—he only wanted to work on his dreams.

It became clear that he needed some physical activity to channel the rhythmic drive that pounded through him. His dreams were filled with images of hand-to-hand combat with inner masculine figures, which I took to mean the unconscious was leading him toward the conscious integration of his chthonic masculine energy—his bull. I suggested he consider a course of Karate or Akido, both highly disciplined, ritualistic forms of Eastern martial arts, but to no avail. I could not even lead his horse to water, let alone make him drink. I could only point out that somewhere out there, there might be a fountain.

Meanwhile, his own instincts were at work. They knew their goal and after exploring several possibilities he himself finally found the right answer: ballroom dancing. He began taking classes two or three times a week, privately as well as in a group. He did this while following a full course of engineering training and, later, holding a full-time job.

This man is a lay dancer. The goddess did not demand that he serve her above all others. Dance, with its careful training and strong rhythmic involvement, disciplined and strengthened his body and greatly reinforced his ego. His strong charge of energy was harnessed, transformed, to serve his needs. His personality became more secure and malleable, and he developed a flexible persona with which to relate to the outside world. Ballroom dancing had the particular advantage of helping him to learn to dance with another person. From the first day he entered analysis his central concern had been to be able to relate to women, and in this too he succeeded—indeed, not long after his foray onto the dance floor he got married. That is what transformation looks like.

Physical training is too time-consuming for an analytic hour. There are, however, many ways of including the body in a session. Close observation of posture, of areas of muscular tension, of localized and general physical activity, facial expressions, etc.— these help to make the ego aware of the body. In addition, the body itself provides a vast source of amplificatory material for translating images from the unconscious into everyday language. But the real body work, the consistent, laborious process of differentiating and awakening the body, needs in my experience to be done separately, outside of the consulting room.

In the physical training arena one learns by doing. In the analytic hour one tries to discover what the doing means psychologically and symbolically. This separation is essential if one is not to become stuck in concrete physicality, if one is to bring the body to consciousness rather than be drowned in its darkness.

Ultimately, if the goal is to become more conscious, physical experience must grow beyond the literal and be turned into psychological knowledge. After one has planted the seed—the tree—in the earth, one must help it reach upward toward the light.

> Here it is the wood that serves as nourishment for the flame, the spirit. All that is visible must grow beyond itself, extend into the realm of the invisible. Thereby it receives its true consecration and clarity and takes firm root in the cosmic order.[3]

---

[3] Richard Wilhelm, trans., *The I Ching or Book of Changes,* Hexagram 50, "The Cauldron," p. 50.

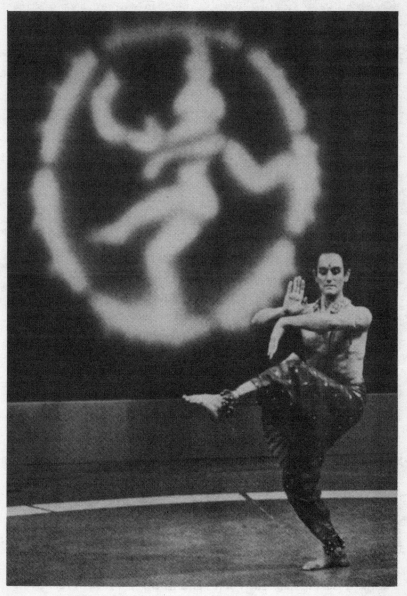
Matteo Vittucci, ethnic dancer and choreographer.

Glossary of Jungian Terms

Active Imagination. A process by which one interacts consciously with contents of the unconscious, through drawing or painting, writing, sculpting, dance, etc.

Anima (Latin, "soul"). The unconscious, feminine side of a man's personality, an inner woman personified in dreams by images ranging from prostitute and seductress to spiritual guide (Sophia). She is the Eros principle in a man's psyche.

Animus (Latin, "spirit"). The unconscious, masculine side of a woman's personality. He personifies the Logos principle. The animus functions in a positive sense as a bridge between the woman's ego and her own creative resources in the unconscious.

Archetypes. Irrepresentable in themselves, but their effects appear in consciousness as archetypal images and ideas, universal patterns or motifs which come from the collective unconscious and are the basic content of religions, mythologies, legends and fairy tales.

Association. The spontaneous flow of interconnected thoughts and images around a specific idea, determined by unconscious connections.

Complex. An emotionally charged group of ideas or images. At the cores of a complex is an archetype or archetypal image (see above).

Coniunctio. The coming together of opposites.

Ego. The central complex in the field of consciousness. A strong ego can relate objectively to activated contents of the unconscious (i.e., other complexes) rather than identifying with them. Identification with a complex appears as a state of possession.

Feeling. One of the four psychic functions in Jung's model of typology. It is a rational function (as is **thinking**) which evaluates the worth of relationships and situations. The feeling function is different from emotional affect, which is due to an activated complex.

114

Individuation. The conscious realization of one's unique psychological reality, including both strengths and limitations. It leads to the experience of the **Self** (see below).

Inflation. A psychological state in which one has an unrealistically high or low (negative inflation) self-image.

Intuition. One of the four psychic functions. It is an irrational function which tells us the possibilities inherent in the present. In contrast to **sensation** (the function which perceives immediate reality through the physical senses), intuition perceives via the unconscious (e.g., flashes of insight of unknown origin).

Mandala. A four-fold structure or image.

Persona (Latin, "actor's mask"). One's social role, derived from the expectations of society and early training.

Projection. The process whereby an unconscious quality or characteristic of one's own is perceived and reacted to in an outer object or person.

Self. The archetype of wholeness and the regulating center of the psyche. It is experienced as a transpersonal power (e.g., God) which transcends the ego.

Shadow. An unconscious part of the personality characterized by traits and attitudes, both positive and negative, which the conscious ego tends to reject or ignore. It is commonly personified in dreams by persons of the same sex as the dreamer.

Symbol. The best possible expression for something essentially unknown. Symbolic thinking is non-linear, right-brain oriented; it is complementary to logical, linear, left-brain thinking.

Transcendent function. The reconciling "third" which emerges from the unconscious in the form of a symbol or a new attitude after conflicting opposites have been held in awareness.

Transference-countertransference. Particular cases of projection, commonly used to described the unconscious, emotional bonds that arise between two persons in a therapeutic relationship.

Bibliography

American Heritage Dictionary. William Morris, ed. Boston: Houghton Mifflin Co., 1969.

Armitage, Merle. *Martha Graham.* Reprint. New York: Dance Horizons, 1966.

Boston Women's Health Book Collective. *Our Bodies, Ourselves.* New York: Simon and Schuster, 1971.

Bührmann, M. Vera. *Living in Two Worlds: Communication Between a White Healer and Her Black Counterparts.* Wilmette, IL: Chiron Publications, 1986.

Cohen, Selma Jeanne, ed. *Doris Humphrey: An Artist First.* Middletown: Wesleyan University Press, 1972.

———. *The Modern Dance: Seven Statements of Belief.* Middletown: Wesleyan University Press, 1965.

Como, William. *Raoul Gelabert's Anatomy for the Dancer.* 2 vols. New York: Dance Magazine, 1964.

Cunningham, Merce. *Changes: Notes on Choreography.* New York: Something Else Press, 1968.

Davidson, H.R. Ellis. *Gods and Myths of Northern Europe.* Middlesex: Penguin Books, 1964.

deMille, Agnes. *Dance to the Piper.* Boston: Little Brown & Co., 1952.

Duncan, Irma. *Duncan Dancer.* Middletown: Wesleyan University Press, 1965.

———. *The Technique of Isadora Duncan.* Reprint. New York: Dance Horizons, 1970.

Duncan, Isadora. *My Life.* New York: Liverwright Press, 1955.

Edinger, Edward F. *Anatomy of the Psyche: Alchemical Symbolism in Psychotherapy.* La Salle, IL: Open Court, 1985.

———. *The Creation of Consciousness: Jung's Myth for Modern Man.* Toronto: Inner City Books, 1984.

———. *Ego and Archetype.* Baltimore: Pelican Books, 1973.

Eliade, Mircea. *Shamanism: Archaic Techniques of Ecstasy* (Bollingen Series LXXVI). Trans. Willard R. Trask. Princeton: Princeton University Press, 1961.

Eliot, T.S. "Burnt Norton," in *Four Quartets*. London: Faber and Faber, 1936.

Emerson, Ralph Waldo. *The Collected Works of Ralph Waldo Emerson,* vol. 3 (Essays: Second Series). Cambridge, MA: Belknap Press, 1983.

Evans, Richard I. *Conversations with Carl Jung*. Princeton: Van Nostrand Co., 1964.

Feinstein Martin, ed. *Martha Graham Dance Company*. Souvenir Program. New York: Hurok Publications, 1966.

Fergusson, Erna. *Dancing Gods: Indian Ceremonies of New Mexico and Arizona*. Albuquerque: University of New Mexico Press, 1966.

Fonteyn, Margot. *Autobiography*. New York: Alfred A. Knopf, 1976.

Frazer, James G. *The Golden Bough*. Abridged ed. New York: Macmillan, 1951.

Graham, Martha. *The Notebooks of Martha Graham*. New York: Harcourt Brace Jovanovich, 1973.

Graves, Robert. *The Greek Myths*. 2 vols. Baltimore: Penguin Books, 1955.

Hamilton, Edith. *Mythology*. Boston: Little Brown & Co., 1942.

Hannah, Barbara. *Encounters with the Soul: Active Imagination as Developed by C.G. Jung*. Santa Monica: Sigo Press, 1981.

_____. *Jung: His Life and Work*. New York: G.P. Putnam's Sons, 1976.

_____. *Striving Towards Wholeness*. New York: G.P. Putnam's Sons, 1971.

Harding, Esther. *Psychic Energy: Its Source and its Transformation* (Bollingen Series X). 2nd. ed. Princeton: Princeton University Press, 1963.

_____. *The Way of All Women*. New York: G.P. Putnam's Sons, 1970.

_____. *Woman's Mysteries*. New York: G.P. Putnam's Sons, 1971.

Humphrey, Doris. *The Art of Making Dances*. New York: Grove Press, Inc., 1959.

Jung, C.G. *The Collected Works* (Bollingen Series XX). 20 vols. Trans. R. F. C. Hull. Ed. H. Read, M. Fordham, G. Adler, Wm. McGuire. Princeton: Princeton University Press, 1953-1979.

_____. *Kundalini Yoga*. In *Spring 1975* (Lectures 1 & 2) and *Spring 1976* (Lectures 3 & 4).

_____. *Letters* (Bollingen Series XCV). 2 vols. Princeton: Princeton University Press, 1973.

_____. *Man and His Symbols*. New York: Doubleday & Co., 1968.

_____. *Memories, Dreams, Reflections*. New York: Pantheon Books, 1961.

_____. *Modern Man in Search of a Soul*. Trans. W.S. Dell and Cary F. Baynes. New York: Harcourt Brace & Co., 1933.

_____. *Nietzsche's Zarathustra* (Bollingen Series XCIX). 2 vols. Ed. James L. Jarrett. Princeton: Princeton University Press, 1988.

_____. *The Visions Seminars*. 2 vols. Zurich: Spring Publications, 1976.

Jung, Emma, and von Franz, Marie-Louise. *The Grail Legend*. Trans. Andrea Dykes. 2nd ed. Boston: Sigo Press, 1986.

Kahn, Fritz. *The Human Body*. New York: Random House, 1965.

Kendall, Elizabeth. *Where She Danced*. New York: Alfred A. Knopf, 1979.

Larousse Encyclopedia of Mythology. New York: Prometheus Press, 1959.

Leatherman, Le Roy, and Swope, Martha. *Martha Graham: Portrait of a Lady as an Artist*. New York: Alfred A. Knopf, 1966.

Lilly, John C. *The Center of the Cyclone: An Autobiography of Inner Space*. New York: Bantam Press, 1972.

Lowen, Alexander. *The Betrayal of the Body*. New York: Collier Books, 1969.

Lyle, Cynthia. *Dancers on Dancing (A Book of Interviews)*. New York: Sterling Publishing Co., Inc., 1977.

Magriel, Paul, ed. *Isadora Duncan*. New York: Henry Holt & Co., 1947.

Martin, John. *John Martin's Book of the Dance*. New York: Tudor Publishing Co., 1963.

_____. *The Modern Dance*. New York: Dance Horizons, 1965.

Maynard, Olga. *American Modern Dancers.* Boston: Little Brown, 1965.

Mazo, Joseph H. *Prime Movers: The Makers of Modern Dance in America.* New York: William Morrow & Co., Inc., 1977.

McDonagh, Don. *Martha Graham.* New York: Prager, 1973.

McNeely, Deldon Anne. *Touching: Body Therapy and Depth Psychology.* Toronto: Inner City Books, Toronto, 1987.

Mensendieck, Bess. *Look Better, Feel Better.* New York: Harper Bros., 1954.

Morgan, Barbara. *Martha Graham: Sixteen Dances in Photographs.* Revised ed. Dobbs Ferry: Morgan & Morgan, 1980.

Neumann, Erich. *The Great Mother* (Bollingen Series XLVII). 2nd ed. Trans. Ralph Manheim. Princeton: Princeton University Press, 1972.

_____. "The Moon and Matriarchal Consciousness." In *Fathers and Mothers.* Zurich: Spring Publications, 1973.

_____. *The Origins and History of Consciousness* (Bollingen Series XLII). Trans. R.F.C. Hull. New York: Pantheon, 1954.

Onians, Richard B. *The Origins of European Thought.* Reprint. New York: The Arno Press, 1973.

Otto, Walter F. *Dionysus: Myth and Cult.* Trans. R.B. Palmer. Bloomington: Indiana University Press, 1965.

_____. *Menschengestalt und Tanz.* München: Hermann Rinn Verlag, 1956.

Pritchard, James B., ed. *The Ancient Near East,* vol. 1. Princeton: Princeton University Press, 1958.

Purce, Jill. *The Mystic Spiral: Journey of the Soul.* New York: Avon Books, 1974.

Rose, Stephen, producer. *A Touch of Sensitivity.* Broadcast transcript. Boston: WGBH-TV, 1980.

Sachs, Curt. *World History of the Dance.* Trans. Bessie Schönberg. New York: W.W. Norton, 1937.

Sechehaye, Marguerite. *Autobiography of a Schizophrenic Girl.* New York: Signet Books, 1970.

Siegel, Marcia. *Watching the Dance Go By.* Boston: Houghton Mifflin Co., 1977.

Snyder, James. *Medieval Art.* New York: Harry N. Abrams, Inc., 1989.

Sorel, Walter, ed. and trans. *The Mary Wigman Book.* Middletown: Wesleyan University Press, 1966.

St. Denis, Ruth. *An Unfinished Life.* New York: Harper Bros., 1939.

van der Post, Laurens. *A Mantis Carol.* New York: William Morrow & Co., 1976.

von Franz, Marie-Louise. *A Psychological Study of the Golden Ass of Apuleius.* New York: Spring Publications, 1970.

_____. *C.G. Jung: His Myth in Our Time.* Trans. William H. Kennedy, New York: G.P. Putnam's Sons, 1975.

_____. *The Feminine in Fairy Tales.* New York: Spring Publications, 1972.

_____. *Number and Time.* Trans. William H. Kennedy. Evanston: Northwestern University Press, 1974.

_____. *Projection and Re-Collection in Jungian Psychology: Reflections of the Soul.* Trans. William H. Kennedy. La Salle, Il: Open Court, 1980.

_____. *Time: Rhythm and Repose.* London: Thames and Hudson, 1978.

Wigman, Mary. *The Language of Dance.* Trans. Walter Sorel. Middletown: Wesleyan University Press, 1966.

Wilhelm, Richard, trans. *The I Ching or Book of Changes* (Bollingen Series XIX). 3rd ed. Trans. into English by Cary F. Baynes. Princeton: Princeton University Press, 1967.

Woodman, Marion. *Addiction to Perfection: The Still Unravished Bride.* Toronto: Inner City Books, 1982.

_____. *The Owl Was a Baker's Daughter: Obesity, Anorexia Nervosa and the Repressed Feminine.* Toronto: Inner City Books, 1980.

_____. *The Pregnant Virgin: A Process of Psychological Transformation.* Toronto: Inner City Books, 1985.

Wosien, Maria-Gabriele. *The Sacred Dance: Encounter with the Gods.* London: Thames and Hudson, 1974.

Zimmer, Heinrich. *Myths and Symbols in Indian Art and Civilization* (Bollingen Series VI). Ed. Joseph Campbell. Princeton: Princeton University Press, 1974.

Index

Numbers in italics refer to illustrations

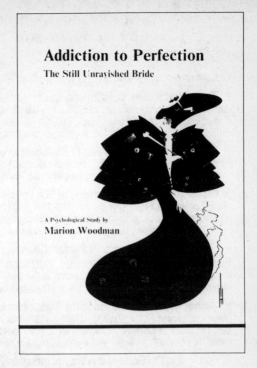

Addiction to Perfection
The Still Unravished Bride

A Psychological Study by
Marion Woodman

12. Addiction to Perfection: The Still Unravished Bride.
Marion Woodman (Toronto). ISBN 0-919123-11-2. 208 pp. $15

"This book is about taking the head off an evil witch." With these words Marion Woodman begins her spiral journey, a powerful and authoritative look at the psychology and attitudes of modern woman.

The witch is a Medusa or a Lady Macbeth, an archetypal pattern functioning autonomously in women, petrifying their spirit and inhibiting their development as free and creatively receptive individuals. Much of this, according to the author, is due to a cultural one-sidedness that favors patriarchal values—productivity, goal orientation, intellectual excellence, spiritual perfection, etc.—at the expense of more earthy, interpersonal values that have traditionally been recognized as the heart of the feminine.

Marion Woodman's first book, *The Owl Was a Baker's Daughter: Obesity, Anorexia Nervosa and the Repressed Feminine*, focused on the psychology of eating disorders and weight disturbances.

Here, with a broader perspective on the same general themes, she continues her remarkable exploration of women's mysteries through case material, dreams, literature and mythology, in food rituals, rape symbolism, Christianity, imagery in the body, sexuality, creativity and relationships.

"It is like finding the loose end in a knotted mass of thread. . . . What a relief! Somebody knows!"—**Elizabeth Strahan,** *Psychological Perspectives.*

Studies in Jungian Psychology
by Jungian Analysts

Limited Edition Paperbacks

Prices and payment in U.S. dollars (except for Canadian orders)

1. The Secret Raven: Conflict and Transformation.
Daryl Sharp (Toronto). ISBN 0-919123-00-7. 128 pp. $13
A practical study of *puer* psychology, including dream interpretation and material on midlife crisis, the provisional life, the mother complex, anima and shadow. Illustrated.

2. The Psychological Meaning of Redemption Motifs in Fairytales.
Marie-Louise von Franz (Zurich). ISBN 0-919123-01-5. 128 pp. $13
Unique approach to understanding typical dream motifs (bathing, clothes, animals, etc.).

3. On Divination and Synchronicity: The Psychology of Meaningful Chance.
Marie-Louise von Franz (Zurich). ISBN 0-919123-02-3. 128 pp. $13
Penetrating study of irrational methods of divining fate (I Ching, astrology, palmistry, Tarot cards, etc.), contrasting Western ideas with those of so-called primitives. Illustrated.

4. The Owl Was a Baker's Daughter: Obesity, Anorexia and the Repressed Feminine. Marion Woodman (Toronto). ISBN 0-919123-03-1. 144 pp. $14
A modern classic, with particular attention to the body as mirror of the psyche in weight disturbances and eating disorders. Based on case studies, dreams and mythology. Illus.

5. Alchemy: An Introduction to the Symbolism and the Psychology.
Marie-Louise von Franz (Zurich). ISBN 0-919123-04-X. 288 pp. $18
Detailed guide to what the alchemists were really looking for: emotional wholeness. Invaluable for interpreting images and motifs in modern dreams and drawings. 84 illustrations.

6. Descent to the Goddess: A Way of Initiation for Women.
Sylvia Brinton Perera (New York). ISBN 0-919123-05-8. 112 pp. $12
A timely and provocative study of the need for an inner, female authority in a masculine-oriented society. Rich in insights from mythology and the author's analytic practice.

7. The Psyche as Sacrament: C.G. Jung and Paul Tillich.
John P. Dourley (Ottawa). ISBN 0-919123-06-6. 128 pp. $13
Comparative study from a dual perspective (author is Catholic priest and Jungian analyst), exploring the psychological meaning of religion, God, Christ, the spirit, the Trinity, etc.

8. Border Crossings: Carlos Castaneda's Path of Knowledge.
Donald Lee Williams (Boulder). ISBN 0-919123-07-4. 160 pp. $14
The first thorough psychological examination of the Don Juan novels, bringing Castaneda's spiritual journey down to earth. Special attention to the psychology of the feminine.

9. Narcissism and Character Transformation. The Psychology of Narcissistic Character Disorders. ISBN 0-919123-08-2. 192 pp. $15
Nathan Schwartz-Salant (New York).
A comprehensive study of narcissistic character disorders, drawing upon a variety of analytic points of view (Jung, Freud, Kohut, Klein, etc.). Theory and clinical material. Illus.

10. Rape and Ritual: A Psychological Study.
Bradley A. Te Paske (Minneapolis). ISBN 0-919123-09-0. 160 pp. $14
Incisive combination of theory, clinical material and mythology. Illustrated.

11. Alcoholism and Women: The Background and the Psychology.
Jan Bauer (Montreal). ISBN 0-919123-10-4. 144 pp. $14
Sociology, case material, dream analysis and archetypal patterns from mythology.

12. Addiction to Perfection: The Still Unravished Bride.
Marion Woodman (Toronto). ISBN 0-919123-11-2. 208 pp. $15
A powerful and authoritative look at the psychology of modern women. Examines dreams, mythology, food rituals, body imagery, sexuality and creativity. A continuing best-seller since its original publication in 1982. Illustrated.

13. Jungian Dream Interpretation: A Handbook of Theory and Practice.
James A. Hall, M.D. (Dallas). ISBN 0-919123-12-0. 128 pp. $13
A practical guide, including common dream motifs and many clinical examples.

14. The Creation of Consciousness: Jung's Myth for Modern Man.
Edward F. Edinger, M.D. (Los Angeles). ISBN 0-919123-13-9. 128 pp. $13
Insightful study of the meaning and purpose of human life. Illustrated.

15. The Analytic Encounter: Transference and Human Relationship.
Mario Jacoby (Zurich). ISBN 0-919123-14-7. 128 pp. $13
Sensitive exploration of the difference between relationships based on projection and
I-Thou relationships characterized by mutual respect and psychological objectivity.

16. Change of Life: Psychological Study of Dreams and the Menopause.
Ann Mankowitz (Santa Fe). ISBN 0-919123-15-5. 128 pp. $13
A moving account of an older woman's Jungian analysis, dramatically revealing the later
years as a time of rebirth, a unique opportunity for psychological development.

17. The Illness That We Are: A Jungian Critique of Christianity.
John P. Dourley (Ottawa). ISBN 0-919123-16-3. 128 pp. $13
Radical study by Catholic priest and analyst, exploring Jung's qualified appreciation of
Christian symbols and ritual, while questioning the masculine ideals of Christianity.

18. Hags and Heroes: A Feminist Approach to Jungian Therapy with Couples.
Polly Young-Eisendrath (Philadelphia). ISBN 0-919123-17-1. 192 pp. $15
Highly original integration of feminist views with the concepts of Jung and Harry Stack
Sullivan. Detailed strategies and techniques, emphasis on feminine authority.

19. Cultural Attitudes in Psychological Perspective.
Joseph Henderson , M.D. (San Francisco). ISBN 0-919123-18-X. 128 pp. $13
Shows how a psychological attitude can give depth to one's world view. Illustrated.

20. The Vertical Labyrinth: Individuation in Jungian Psychology.
Aldo Carotenuto (Rome). ISBN 0-919123-19-8. 144 pp. $14
A guided journey through the world of dreams and psychic reality, illustrating the process
of individual psychological development.

21. The Pregnant Virgin: A Process of Psychological Transformation.
Marion Woodman (Toronto). ISBN 0-919123-20-1. 208 pp. $16
A celebration of the feminine, in both men and women. Explores the wisdom of the body,
eating disorders, relationships, dreams, addictions, etc. Illustrated.

22. Encounter with the Self: William Blake's *Illustrations of the Book of Job.*
Edward F. Edinger, M.D. (Los Angeles). ISBN 0-919123-21-X. 80 pp. $10
Penetrating commentary on the Biblical Job story as a numinous, archetypal event.
Complete with Blake's original 22 engravings.

23. The Scapegoat Complex: Toward a Mythology of Shadow and Guilt.
Sylvia Brinton Perera (New York). ISBN 0-919123-22-8. 128 pp. $13
A hard-hitting study of victim psychology in modern men and women, based on case
material, mythology and archetypal patterns.

24. The Bible and the Psyche: Individuation Symbolism in the Old Testament.
Edward F. Edinger (Los Angeles). ISBN 0-919123-23-6. 176 pp. $15
A major new work relating significant Biblical events to the psychological movement
toward wholeness that takes place in individuals.

25. The Spiral Way: A Woman's Healing Journey.
Aldo Carotenuto (Rome). ISBN 0-919123-24-4. 144 pp. $14
Detailed case history of a fifty-year-old woman's Jungian analysis, with particular attention
to her dreams and the rediscovery of her enthusiasm for life.

26. The Jungian Experience: Analysis and Individuation.
James A. Hall, M.D. (Dallas). ISBN 0-919123-25-2. 176 pp. $15
Comprehensive study of the theory and clinical application of Jungian thought, including
Jung's model, the structure of analysis, where to find an analyst, training centers, etc.

27. Phallos: Sacred Image of the Masculine.
Eugene Monick (Scranton/New York). ISBN 0-919123-26-0. 144 pp. $14
Uncovers the essence of masculinity (as opposed to the patriarchy) through close examination of the physical, mythological and psychological aspects of phallos. **30 illustrations.**

28. The Christian Archetype: A Jungian Commentary on the Life of Christ.
Edward F. Edinger, M.D. (Los Angeles). ISBN 0-919123-27-9. 144 pp. $14
Psychological view of images and events central to the Christian myth, showing their symbolic meaning in terms of personal individuation. **31 illustrations.**

29. Love, Celibacy and the Inner Marriage.
John P. Dourley (Ottawa). ISBN 0-919123-28-7. 128 pp. $13
Shows that without a deeply compassionate relationship to the inner anima/animus, we cannot relate to our intimates or to God, to the full depth of our ability to love.

30. Touching: Body Therapy and Depth Psychology.
Deldon Anne McNeely (Lynchburg, VA). ISBN 0-919123-29-5. 128 pp. $13
Illustrates how these two disciplines, both concerned with restoring life to an ailing human psyche, may be integrated in theory and practice. Focus on the healing power of touch.

31. Personality Types: Jung's Model of Typology.
Daryl Sharp (Toronto). ISBN 0-919123-30-9. 128 pp. $13
Detailed explanation of Jung's model (basis for the widely-used Myers-Briggs Type Indicator), showing its implications for individual development and for relationships. Illus.

32. The Sacred Prostitute: Eternal Aspect of the Feminine.
Nancy Qualls-Corbett (Birmingham). ISBN 0-919123-31-7. 176 pp. $15
Shows how our vitality and capacity for joy depend on rediscovering the ancient connection between spirituality and passionate love. Illustrated. **(Foreword by Marion Woodman.)**

33. When the Spirits Come Back.
Janet O. Dallett (Seal Harbor, WA). ISBN 0-919123-32-5. 160 pp. $14
An analyst examines herself, her profession and the limitations of prevailing attitudes toward mental disturbance. Interweaving her own story with descriptions of those who come to her for help, she details her rediscovery of the integrity of the healing process.

34. The Mother: Archetypal Image in Fairy Tales.
Sibylle Birkhäuser-Oeri (Zurich). ISBN 0-919123-33-3. 176 pp. $15
Compares processes in the unconscious with common images and motifs in folk-lore. Illustrates how positive and negative mother complexes affect us all, with examples from many well-known fairy tales and daily life. **(Edited by Marie-Louise von Franz.)**

35. The Survival Papers: Anatomy of a Midlife Crisis.
Daryl Sharp (Toronto). ISBN 0-919123-34-1. 160 pp. $15
Jung's major concepts—persona, shadow, anima and animus, complexes, projection, typology, active imagination, individuation, etc.—are dramatically presented in the immediate context of an analysand's process. And the analyst's.

36. The Cassandra Complex: Living with Disbelief.
Laurie Layton Schapira (New York). ISBN 0-919123-35-X. 160 pp. $15
Shows how unconscious, prophetic sensibilities can be transformed from a burden into a valuable source of conscious understanding. Includes clinical material and an examination of the role of powerfully intuitive, medial women through history. Illustrated.

37. Dear Gladys: The Survival Papers, Book 2
Daryl Sharp (Toronto). ISBN 0-919123-36-8. 144 pp. $15
An entertaining and instructive continuation of the story begun in *The Survival Papers* (title 35). Part textbook, part novel, part personal exposition.

Prices and payment (check or money order) in $U.S. (in Canada, $Cdn)

Please add $1 per book (bookpost) or $3 per book (airmail)

INNER CITY BOOKS
Box 1271, Station Q, Toronto, Canada M4T 2P4